"At the core of Kevin's coaching is the audacious notion that just as one can lace up shoes with the goal of running six miles, one can lace up with the goal of mindfully drawing energy from the run and arriving at the finish with surplus peace of mind and focus. In Kevin's system, as outlined in *The Heart of Running*, our physical, mental, and spiritual aspects are treated as intrinsic and inseparable, but also—and this is the important part—trainable."

—BART LONGACRE
Social Sciences Computing Services Manager at the
University of Chicago and Triathlete

"The MQ, as Kevin Everett describes in his *The Heart of Running*, can be used in all activities of life, not just with athletics. I've enjoyed applying it to my other passion, which is horseback riding. The MQ has even increased my body awareness during more mundane activities such as grocery shopping, house cleaning, mowing the lawn, etc."

—JANINE FRANCO
Physician Assistant and Triathlete

"No matter who you are or where you are at in your running journey, the concepts in *The Heart of Running* will help you achieve your goals and enable you to run farther, longer, healthier, and happier! It doesn't get much better than that!"

—JENN HALLADAY
Multiple winner of 200+ mile Lotoja Classic Cycling race

"This book has changed my running! I used to run to count the miles, now I enjoy my time spent running. My running has become meaningful and focused; yet easier. It's an entirely different experience for me. I will be running for the rest of my life using this plan! Focusing on my breathing, being mindful of each step, and balancing my body has made a huge difference. Whether you are an experienced or novice runner, this book is a must-read! It will elevate and improve your running!"

—SHARYN BARRETT
R.N. and Triathlete

"Although I consider myself a runner, I have never felt like I was achieving my optimum performance. Embracing the knowledge in *The Heart of Running* will allow you not only to enjoy running, but to reach your ultimate goal: the Runner's High."

—NATALIE SHIFLETT
M.D., 10-time Ironman finisher, All World Athlete

"In *The Heart of Running*, Kevin Everett has been able to put into words what every runner wishes to achieve. By applying his principles of kinesthetic awareness, you can become not only a better runner, but a better athlete in general. He takes you on an amazing journey to show you how your mind and body become one."

—BRYAN SHIFLETT
M.D., 9-time Kona qualifier, All World Athlete

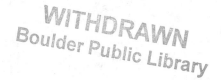
PRAISE FOR
THE HEART OF RUNNING

"With all the books on running, I sometimes wonder what more there is to say. Well, Kevin Everett has a lot of new insight in his indispensable book, *The Heart Of Running*. It's for runners, non-runners, and those who may become runners or will just include movement in their lives. Everett is an expert of motion in every conceivable way. He shows us how to make motion a part of our daily lives. Let him help you get moving!"

—GEORGE HIRSCH
Former Publisher of *Runner's World Magazine*

"I have had the privilege of having Kevin coach me through two Ironman races. His philosophy of exercise as empowered play has truly changed the sport for me in such a positive way. *The Heart of Running* not only will help you become a better athlete, but also a happier athlete."

—CHRISTINE TURPIN
Mother and Triathlete

"*The Heart of Running* is a brilliant combination of running science and real-life wisdom. Kevin Everett possesses the secret to living a fuller, happier, and healthier life and is revolutionary in leading us to our highest potential. As the mother of five children, having a family business, and being a part-time personal trainer, marathoner, and triathlete, I have little time and energy. I used to approach running as a task and "muscled" my way through training and races. The MQ have altered my mindset and every motion. By first truly learning to walk, and recruiting all my available power, I have gained strength, coordination, agility, speed, and stamina. My son feels empowered and can run longer, stronger, and faster as he competes in high school cross country. Kevin provided the tools for him to engage every part of his body and make every step count. I feel aware and energized in all my motions: running, swimming, biking, and even doing household chores. I now walk down the aisles of the grocery store with swagger!"

—CONNIE MCMURRAY
Business Owner, Part-time Personal Trainer,
Marathoner, and Triathlete

"Kevin Everett participates in running much like dancers approach their craft—as an art form. He brings a wisdom and mindfulness to his approach that elevate the mechanics and athletics of the sport to a new level—one that is about creating good and not just 'winning.'"

—JOHN MICHAEL SCHERT
Artist, Producer, and Social Entrepreneur

"I love running! I have had the opportunity to train with and be mentored by Kevin Everett. The knowledge and methodology developed and discussed in *The Heart of Running* have helped me become so much more aware of what I am actually doing while I run. I can run pretty well, but I am just realizing what my potential can be because of what they have taught me. This is a lifetime sport and I am so excited to keep learning. This book is just the beginning of an incredible journey!"

—**LEXY HALLADAY**
High School Freshman Runner (4:46 mile)

"As an athlete, walking has been a part of my life each and every day, yet I had never thought about how I walked. It was just an instinctual habit. Now, with the help of Kevin Everett's *The Heart of Running* and MQ, the way I walk has made me mindful of how my body moves. MQ has brought a new meaning to every aspect of my life."

—**SPENCER FERRER**
High School Senior and Mountain Biker

"*The Heart of Running* takes what some many consider only a sport of fitness and allows the reader to embark on a journey that enriches the mind and inspires the soul. It is beautifully written and filled with practical application for the runner and life enthusiast."

—**BRADY MURRAY**
CFP®President/CEO at MassMutual Financial Group—
Intermountain West and Triathlete

"What if the art in the heart of running is all about walking? What if walking lays the foundation for something more to happen? What if walking is the most important door to open to discover mastery of all human motions?" This quote from *The Heart of Running*, by Kevin Everett, is the foundation for his innovative approach to understanding how simply walking with proper MQ: motion, mindfulness, and meaning, can bring about monumental positive results in well-being, awareness, and health in all activities of your life.

"I heartily recommend this book for anyone who wants to connect their heart, mind, and physical activity together for positive life changes."

—KAREN MORRISON
Director, AquAbility

"*The Heart of Running* brings to light the concept of flow in our daily life. In a world where the norm is to compartmentalize and strive for balance, this speaks to the concept of creating a life where we feel a sense of connection of each life element. Striving to change our perception of the moment we are in—and why—can bring a fresh sense of meaning to the role that being a runner plays in life and the simple act of running."

—MARNI MCDOWELL
M.S., R.D. Global Team Member Programs Manager at Micron

"*The Heart of Running* has so much heart and is so empowering that I was in a state of flow just reading it! Kevin Everett has provided such a clear and meaningful discussion of how we can fall in love with running—or fall in love again after a long struggle with the return. Everett provides a way to begin a personal journey 'toward a deeper understanding of how and why to run well.' This is not easy to communicate or to do, yet Everett does both so well. Truly, the book is a guide for how to thrive."

—CATHY BROAD
Lawyer, Triathlete, and Yoga Instructor

"*The Heart of Running* is more like a mantra than a manual. Kevin Everett uses running as a way for readers to seek a higher level of consciousness, not only in athletics, but in their day-to-day lives. He uses the analytical mind of a swimmer to codify efficient running technique with a unique introspective approach that leaves no stone unturned. As a high school cross country coach and former professional triathlete, I can safely say that *The Heart of Running* is equally relevant to both new and experienced runners."

—CHRIS FOSTER
Professional Triathlete and Freelance Writer

THE
HEART
OF
RUNNING

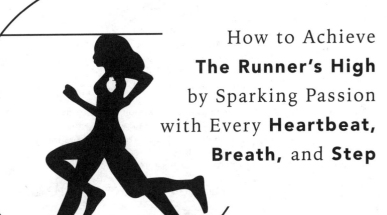

How to Achieve
The Runner's High
by Sparking Passion
with Every **Heartbeat,**
Breath, and **Step**

KEVIN EVERETT

Published in Boise, Idaho by Elevate. An imprint of Elevate Publishing.

This book may be purchased in bulk for educational, business, organizational, or promotional use.

For information, please email info@elevatepub.com

Paperback ISBN-13: 9781943425914

eBook ISBN-13: 9781943425921

Library of Congress Control Number: 2016942584

Printed in the United States of America.

AWAKEN THE
RUNNING SPIRIT

The heart of running is a choice; it is an awareness. A way of being. Being aware. An ancient concept known as Satori is one way to illustrate it. This book will show you paths toward achieving a Runner's High on every outing. It is simple, yet not easy. A Runner's High is a discovery of a flow state. A flow state is the highest level of being where you feel and perform at your best. It is the edge you seek. It is the purpose you need. It is the heart of running. It is the heart of any activity. This book takes running as a catalyst to discuss the potential paths to this wondrous state you can all achieve with one aware breath.

TABLE OF **CONTENTS**

FOREWORD..I

PUBLISHER'S PREFACE..V

AUTHOR'S NOTE..IX

ACKNOWLEDGMENTS...XV

A BEGINNER'S MIND..1

REASONS FOR RUNNING.................................. 15

COACHING AS PLAY..35

EATING WITH HEARTFULNESS............................51

MEASURE YOUR WELL-BEING (MQ)....................71

BREATHING AS A BRIDGE

    A.   TO THE SOUL...103
    B.   TO THE BODY..115

MIND YOUR POSTURE..131

THE POWER OF BALANCE...................................143

HEALING IS A CHOICE...171

THE BEAUTY OF TIMING.....................................191

ABOUT THE AUTHOR...211

WHAT IS **SATORI?**

One definition: "Seeing your true nature or essence."
Another: The highest awareness.

Okay, what is our essence/highest awareness?
LOVE!

The greatest intelligence is the intelligence of the heart.

In the process of becoming a better runner,
the true gift is becoming a better human.

Spark passion for every breath
and every step.

DEDICATION

To all the future runners of the world: may they know and appreciate the paths they embark, creating a world that expands on the discovery of the human heart.

FOREWORD

To experience the perfection and beauty of a Runner's High—a state of flow in a conscious state where you feel your best and perform your best—is to be at a loss for words. If you have felt it, you know the appeal. For those who have not, you have heard the lore. Science has even verified it. *The Heart of Running* is a teaching about the essence of running. At the core of running is something simple, basic, and pure that lies within each of us. This teaching will start you on a journey to find it, to know your running, and perhaps to know yourself in the process.

To know your running, you will first need to understand the blending of the physical with the metaphysical. This teaching will mirror this inner reflection by contrasting the physical connections of the body and mind with the metaphysical relationships of the mind and soul. The mind's gift is its ability to connect these two realms, to act as the bonding agent for the body and soul. The mind is a bridge. In this process, relationships can be explored from different perspectives and a deeper understanding of something as simple as the breath can be known.

To know your running will take balance in your running, balance in your relationships, and balance in your life. This teaching aims to take one possible path of many to discover the true runner inside you. Not just to be a good runner but a good person too. By finding meaning and purpose in your running, it is only a small leap to find meaning and purpose in life. It is a path to knowing yourself. By understanding the internal affairs, consider the dialogue of the body and mind while running; the trust and the love that must take place to run well can leap into every action. Running is a path towards knowing yourself on a deeper, more nuanced level.

Knowledge is with You. Where are You?

This teaching will address the running technique innate to all of you. While it is simple and basic, it will start you on a journey toward a deeper understanding of how and why to run well. While simple and basic, it is a teaching of the highest orders of not just being a good runner but also finding meaning and purpose through your relationships. Running just happens to be one path of thousands that can illustrate this point.

The information age has helped a generation become aware that humans are not just good runners, but extraordinary endurance runners. Yet this natural gift is far from being utilized in today's world. You are a superhero with profound abilities, but, for many, these abilities are hidden. There is a parallel to draw from this for those who lose touch with their meaning and purpose. Just like it is an easy argument to state, "Society is turning blind eyes to its natural gift of endurance."

This is a teaching to know your running. To know it from every angle. To have this level of awareness means achieving a Runner's High every time you run. While this teaching can highlight some steps and open some doors, you will have to take those steps, practice those steps, and run through the doors that are opened. Any book can only open a door, a door you must pass through and experience. The journey is exhilarating, profound, and mysterious. *The journey starts by taking a first breath and knowing where it leads.* The aim of this teaching is to take the true experience you know as a Runner's High and expand it into every breath you take, not just in running but in life.

The first step of a grand journey begins with your first aware breath.

A Runner's High is nothing more than being in a state of flow, a high level of consciousness that feels great. Runners will tap into this state and experience moments of awe—perhaps just seconds before they are exhausted and break down their form. Then, something clicks, time slows down, energy flows, and the speed feels effortless. The first experience is magical and fleeting. Some will spend a lifetime chasing it, wrongly thinking they need to run harder, longer, and faster to achieve it. It is much simpler than that; you simply must pay attention. There can be no distractions; it must be a total and complete awareness of the running body—a body, mind, and heart all running in sync and pulsing as one. A whole body running. Wholeheartedly running. Running with heart. You are not "doing" running; you are being the runner.

True running, running true, running with truth, running in truth, truth in running, and truth with running. This is beautiful running, an alignment that harmonizes your movement. A symmetry in motion. A clarity for each breath and each step stemming from being centered. Being centered. Be centered. This goes beyond balance and into the realm of your entire Being. You see, to achieve your potential in running, you will need to be centered not just in your physical balance but also in your spiritual balance. This means grasping your purpose. It helps to know your middle point. The point of balance in the outer and inner world. Your sacred neutral. The heart is the key to the sacred neutral. This is where true understanding happens. In this space of the heart, all is even, everything simply is. All is love. Having this alignment will amplify you. This is why you will notice sacred geometry throughout this book.

Sacred geometry is truth and simplicity. The middle point creates symmetry that speaks to you on a deeper level of understanding. Sacred geometry is simple, and yet mastering it will take a lifetime. It is in this relationship of playing with simple concepts that seeds for growth are planted. When you look at art, one of the potential gifts is the opening of your heart. The work calms you in a way, allowing the pools of the mind to be still and reflective, and opens a gateway to the heart. Sacred geometry is true balance, symmetry, and centeredness, the same alignment you seek in your running. The same alignment YOU seek.

PUBLISHER'S PREFACE

Why we published *The Heart of Running*

In 2008, Laurie and I launched our publishing company. In the early years, we worked endlessly securing authors, editing, mailing, marketing, and everything in between. Years later, at the age of 39, I found I wasn't satisfied with my life. I worked too much and played too little. I had gained weight and felt directionless.

That summer my kids, Noah and Anastasia, joined the triathlon summer program at our local YMCA. When I was 12 years old, I had watched one of my father's colleagues compete in a triathlon and was instantly engaged. I had always wanted to become a triathlete. But I never did.

It was a dream consumed not only by the craziness of life, but also by a long list of excuses.

I was always too busy and didn't have a good bike. What if I couldn't survive the swim? What if I did manage the swim, only to lose steam in the run? My worries were endless.

Even still, the dream to be a triathlete lived deep within my soul.

Anastasia and Noah flourished that summer. I saw the

transformation in their bodies as they became fit and muscular from all the triathlon playing. I longed to be a kid again. But I assumed my day had passed.

During this time, I got to know Kevin, an amazing and impressive professional triathlete, who could swim faster, bike faster, and run faster than anyone I had ever known. He was also the head coach of the kids triathlon program.

Despite his intensity and obvious competitiveness, Kevin was a kind and gentle soul, who valued family and clearly cared about kids. He wasn't intimidating and, over time, convinced me that I not only could compete in a triathlon, but would live to tell others about it afterward.

Slowly, I started to get in shape. Within a few months, I found myself at the starting line of my first triathlon. I swam 750 yards in 18 minutes and 50 seconds—good enough for 211th place out of 231 competitors. But I did survive the swim and, for that matter, the bike and the run. I made it to the finish line. My super-fit peers wondered how my mediocre performance could bring me such joy, such pride. I knew the reason: I had become a triathlete.

Five years later, while still not fast enough to qualify for the Olympics, I can swim faster, bike faster, and run faster than I ever imagined. And I keep getting faster with age.

Without Kevin, I know I'd still be overweight and dreaming of what could have been.

Kevin helped me believe in myself, and he showed me that I could live out my childhood dreams as an overworked adult. He taught me how to play again.

But Kevin didn't only help me, he helped my wife, my kids, my friends, and hundreds of others who have been chasing dreams like mine.

Kevin is an intensely curious person who continues to learn. He has learned anew the importance of walking and breathing correctly. This past year, he transformed how I walk and breathe. Both things I thought I did quite well. But learning these new mechanics have transformed my athletic endeavors and taken me to a new level I never thought imaginable.

Not only is my physical fitness better than ever, the mental, emotional, and professional parts of my life have also reached a new level.

Kevin values the whole person and the whole of life, and that comes through in his coaching and his writing.

The Heart of Running is a journey to living at the next level. That's why we published this book and feel it's important for you to read. Even more than reading, we hope that you will consume it, keep it by your bed, and let it inspire you to keep moving, to keep playing.

Kevin has done all this and more for my family. I hope you allow him to do the same for you and yours.

Run on,

Mark L. Russell, CEO of Elevate Publishing

AUTHOR'S NOTE:

This teaching about understanding the heart of running is knowing a pure experience *so that you can achieve a Runner's High every outing.*

While this book is about running, it is more about the gift of running. Running is simply a tool for knowing yourself. The gift is applying this knowledge in a meaningful and purposeful way to any action.

Purpose is with You. Where are You?

Playing with the forces that help you run well will give you a deeper sense of who you are and how to be.

Running is one of those nets cast out to ensnare souls with an opportunity to take a path for meaning and purpose through self-discovery. A teaching of steps to allow paths to be explored and practiced in a way to know not just your running but YOU.

Wellness is awareness.

Align your thoughts and emotions with a focus that sparks the greatest creative force, a source and a potential that lie within you.

So, what is the heart of running? This text will make the argument a simple one. But remember, *simple* should not be confused with *easy*. While the heart of running is simple to understand, putting it into practice is a lifelong exploration. At the heart of running is awareness. An ancient Japanese term, Satori, illuminates this idea. Satori is the highest level of awareness; it is knowing your true essence. Wellness is awareness, so…be aware.

Energy goes wherever attention flows. Harnessing and harvesting the energy emanating from the heart is a powerful way to run and goes much deeper than what might appear on the surface. It's a way of being in relationships. A way of being in harmony with your Being—mind, body, heart, and soul. This book is about the art of practice to BE the runner.

THIS IS A TEACHING ABOUT YOUR RELATIONSHIP WITH RUNNING.

Many have a relationship *to* running but this is about Being a runner and having a deep and centered relationship *with* running. This program will teach you how to run for your life. Running is one thing; running well is a lifelong quest for deeper levels of awareness in your breath, your balance, your fitness, your form, your relationships, and much more. The process empowers you to obtain a deeper level of fulfillment through your running.

BEFORE WE BEGIN, LET'S SET THE FOUNDATION, THE CODE, FOR *THE HEART OF RUNNING*:

- Cadence = 180 (90 per leg)
- Foot strike happens on the plumb line (over your center of gravity with sound posture)

- The foot is coming backwards before it strikes the plumb line
- Heartfulness (synonymous with mindfulness)
- Balanced breathing
- Activating the rotational forces

Okay, that's it. Ha! If you can master these fundamentals of running, you have the foundation for matching your life span and your health span with running bliss.

The technique is simple, and yet it will take dedication that few have been able to master. But to really know your running, you will need to mix in some "heart and soul." One of the best ways to do this is through the breath. Conscious breathing. It is not about the breath as much as it is about the awareness, the consciousness of the breath. This is the heartfulness aspect, a passion for life and Pure Experience. You will need to cultivate mindfulness. Can you be aware of every foot strike while running? A simple concept and yet few ever grasp the depth of the inquiry.

There is always another path and a yet-revealed route. Utilize a beginner's mind to discover something new on each run whether it's been done 1,000 times or it's your first.

You have a burning desire for fulfillment. This is a fire that you cannot put out. This is a fire that exists in you now. This represents your greater yearning for fulfillment. You all have a "runner" deep down inside waiting for an outlet of expression.

XII   THE HEART OF RUNNING

TRUE RUNNING IS A FORM OF SELF-DISCOVERY. TO KNOW YOURSELF IS TO KNOW YOUR PURPOSE.

Here, a path is offered directly to the greater possibility of knowing the true joys of running by cultivating the great resources within you. No matter your level of running.

Whether you are beginning or consider yourself a master, accept that there is always a way to deepen your understanding of your craft. This is a challenge to begin a journey. An adventure to discover, not just to believe in your running but to know your running. To know your running form from every angle. In this knowing is a way to tap into the source of joy innate in everyone.

The above steps are the code and the "hack" for running like a deer. This is you, beginning to gain all the secrets of knowing your running form. To BE the runner.

THE JOURNEY IS LIFELONG, AND THE PATHS YOU WILL DISCOVER ARE NUMEROUS.

This program will lay out some of these paths. In your mastery of running, you will find more. The places running can take you physically, mentally, and spiritually are boundless.

A few of the well-trotted tracks will be discussed here. It's important to note that by following the code laid out earlier, with time and focus, you will discover these aspects on your own. This teaching can shine a light on a few paths and lend a helping hand to speed up the process. Running with joy is your potential, and you have it in you right now.

As your running partner and guide, the program will take

you on paths to aid you in your process of mastering the code for running, but the real gift is the discovery and understanding—the knowing—of yourself.

This is a teaching about knowing your run through your own exploration. It will illuminate some paths, but you will choose; you will decide how many of the adventurous and mysterious paths you want to discover.

Applying a beginner's mind—deep intentions, the deepest desires that one may have—to run with heart and know yourself is the goal: accessing your true capacity by cultivating awareness for being in touch, in touch with your Being and your essence through practice. In this application of form, each step and each breath can be a new discovery. One aspect to this awareness is using the art of running to exercise your "muscle," which is your concentration and focus for mindfulness.

Running is one path of millions to take for teaching the *Mindful Arts*. To dance with the body, mind, and soul in unison, to be in the moment and let the love affair that is your life unfold. If you want to be better at running, find joy in running, or perhaps master running, you will need to study mindfulness/heartfulness.

Having a Pure Experience—the Runner's High as an example—can be as simple as inhabiting your Being in awareness. Giving yourself fully to the activity of your moment. This teaching will highlight the path of mindfulness through running. The secret will be applying this knowledge gained by opening the door to running with *heart* in every aspect of your life. Each breath you take has the potential to be one with Pure Experience.

This is a teaching about knowing your running, but in doing

this, you may discover more about yourself in the process, and this is the gift. To know your entire life with meaning and purpose for each activity and relationship you encounter. This is an aspect of running for your life…as an expression of compassion for life.

THE HEART OF RUNNING WILL HELP YOU UNCOVER:

- The essence of running
- Self-discovery via running
- The art of running
- Satori running
- The heart and soul of running
- Meditative running
- Running awareness
- How to know your run
- Mindfulness Being
- Aware running
- Meaningful running
- Optimized running
- An understanding of action
- Balanced running
- Sustainable running
- BeRun, LoveRun
- Being the runner
- Running in the moment
- A Pure Experience
- Flow running
- The Runner's High
- Running's inner journey
- Running's path

ACKNOWLEDGMENTS

The genius in the art of *The Heart of Running* came in waves and accumulated over the years into an ocean of awareness. It is born from empathy and the interaction, curiosity, and discovery that can happen with relationships. The stage is set when a coach and mentor team up to take a challenging path. A student will come to a coach, hungry for something more…hungry to get more out of themselves.

We feed and nourish the student with ideas, perspectives, and attitudes. We find the angle for their next step. Day after day, you start to see changes in their thought and emotional process. We hold the student accountable. They begin to have a feeling. Then, it upgrades into a belief. When this mirrors up with awareness, amazing things happen. The transformation is often seamless, happening in small increments daily until together the days add up to a completion of form. Coaching for over two decades, I've witnessed countless transformations, each one powerful in its own way. Witnessing the adaptations take place can be just as powerful for me, as a coach as it is for the student going through the process of change. As coaches, we store each experience in our library to use in creative ways for the next metamorphosis to take shape.

I've been fortunate to work with six year olds and 70 year olds all seeking out their own unique conversion. Witnessing these alterations has had a profound effect, and I'm grateful for seeing how fast people make a change when they decide it's time. I love being a catalyst for setting up serendipity. In the process, I always get coached as well. The synergy is powerful. To illustrate one of these memorable experiences, let's dive into one relationship in particular.

I met Alissa and her boys on April 30th, 2014 after a short exchange of emails. I was the head coach for the local YMCA Triathlon program and she was inquiring about it. Knowing only that Lucas was born with a rare and life-limiting neurological condition and was limited to a wheelchair, I did not see this as a problem, but more as an opportunity and a challenge to find play in one of its many forms.

Triathlon!? For a six-year-old boy confined to a wheelchair, you say? Absolutely!

See the possibilities.

One of the key characteristics of a coach is to see, create, and imagine the best in people.

Alissa, Noah, and Lucas came to the Y and met with me in the "cave" (our TriClub office tucked away nicely in the basement with no windows and lots of endurance equipment). It was striking and immediately noticeable the bond the brothers had. For most other brothers, the closeness would have been crossing personal space boundaries. But these two had a different way of communicating. Lucas has an amazing presence. I'll never forget the smile he had when we first met. It said everything I needed to know about Lucas. The intelligence in his eyes opened up my heart. His eyes are his best source of communication, albeit with the closeness of the brothers I think Noah picks up more than just Lucas's gaze.

I was struck by Noah's poise as well. At only eight, he seemed to have some character values well beyond his years. I recognized the gift of having a younger brother with special needs. Noah has an ability to empathize and be compassionate that envelopes his character.

Lucas has severely impaired motor skills from a disorder known as lissencephaly. The family was there to meet and talk about ways to incorporate Lucas and Noah into our youth triathlon program at the Y.

I knew we could make this work. I wasn't sure exactly what we could do, but I knew it would be a playful journey of discovering the ways we could train. My main objective was to be welcoming and to listen so that we could be supportive of their needs. Then walked in Willie. William Stewart is also known as the legend that he is, "one-arm Willie." Willie is one of my favorite people, and he's taught me so much. He is one of those characters that has experienced a rich life and has energy to give back. He helped convey the possibilities, and I think Willie was the first to recognize that the story had implications at the national level. Shortly after that, another superhero of the TriClub coaching staff came in, Kelly Driver, and the meeting really took on a celebration to start this playful journey. We were all psyched to set the stage for some brotherly play.

The next day, Alissa, Lucas, and Noah came to a TriClub

practice, and we facilitated some play. We found out that Noah had some work to do on his swimming and that with a little help from Alissa, Lucas could participate in all our swim, bike, run activities. I think we had subtly mentioned some racing opportunities in our first meeting but hadn't really locked anything down yet. After a few TriClub practices, we had a summer goal: The Y-Not Triathlon on July 12. That gave the family just two months to get ready for Noah to pull and push Lucas through an entire triathlon. Did I mention Noah couldn't really swim…? That didn't faze Noah; he is brave, determined, and fueled with love for his brother.

I've seen kids transform from barely keeping their heads above water to completing a 150-yard swim in one week. So I was confident Noah would gain the skills he needed to swim in a lake while pulling his brother. But he would need to be committed to weekly practice/play.

Alissa and Noah came to a few of the adult one-hour swim clinics that I coach. For Noah, we mostly just enabled some time to be in the water and play for the first couple sessions. After a few sessions, he was getting confident in the water having learned his balance. The seamless transformation had begun.

The journey was amazing for me; I can only imagine the joy for the Aldrichs. We spent several weeks out biking around downtown Boise meandering down the greenbelt. It felt good to have a family playing together in our program. Sometimes Alissa would pull Lucas in a chariot, and sometimes Noah would show off his strength by taking a turn. Alissa is fortunate to be able to come out and play with her sons, and it brings much joy to see them interact together.

Triathlon is wonderful for creating imaginative ways to get outside and explore as an entire family.

Lucas and Noah completed the triathlon and did it with smiles, just two months after walking into the cave and inquiring about triathlons. Little did we know that the local news coverage was soon going to go viral on an international scale!

Playing a role and seeing a transformation take place is a life-changing event. It is delightful to see the Aldrich family be able to share their story of love and its profound implications with the world.

I'm grateful for getting to know the Aldrichs, and the lesson from two brothers is one I'll never forget! Love manifesting in the power of play. Keep playing Aldrich family; we're just getting warmed up.

Like Newton famously said, we are "standing on the shoulders of giants." We strive to absorb and understand the knowledge passed down from the generations before us and pass it along to meet the standards of the day. Wisdom is learned, and it can be accelerated through relationships so that the knowledge can be applied to today.

I am grateful to all the mentors in my life, those who were direct coaches and those who lead by example. Trial and error is a slow way to learn; sometimes it can be impactful to learn the slow way, but it is more fun to have someone streamline your progress.

My wife is the bee tree flowering with all the nectar that has me flying and drinking from the source of life. Being with her, learning with her, setting our sights together, and growing our understanding of what it means to be fulfilled is a nourishment that empowers me to be my best self.

Together we did something amazing and produced two of the happiest, liveliest little beings on the planet. Our son and daughter are the sweet spice of life, showing us the way moment to moment. Any parent will attest to the evolution of knowledge that caregiving can give, and I am grateful for being such a fortunate father.

My immediate family played an integral role in my character and understanding and purpose in life. My father, mother, and brother illuminated a path for empathy at an early age and laid down a foundation for allowing me to be an impactful coach by utilizing this one prevailing trait.

My extended French family (my wife is French) has given me a beautiful contrast to an American upbringing and given me a fresh perspective on ways to be. Much of the time and space to write this book came while living in France and writing within earshot of 15th-century church bells, reminding me every 30 minutes of how much time had been gained. The support and understanding along with welcoming and accepting their American family member is something I am most grateful for.

I was fortunate to have interacted with many coaches over the years, each sharing a piece of their puzzle with me. Frank Burlison, Pere Hovland, Charles Todd McClune, Sean Peters, Randy Teeters were a few of my swim coaches who set in motion my motion awareness.

Upon graduating college and ending my collegiate swimming

career, I began six years of being a recreational athlete. Mostly water sports like kayaking, water polo, and snowboarding. Then, I challenged myself by jumping into triathlon, turning pro at 30, just two years after beginning to run and bike competitively. I have mentors to thank for this feat, and Thomas L. Coleman Jr., founder of WN Precision 3D Solutions, was huge. He set the stage for me to excel in biking but also in motion. His awareness for motion is off the charts, and he quickly took my biking awareness to the next level and then the next. So much so, that he improved my swimming by introducing me to contralateral behavior on the bike, which eventually rolled into running and walking. Tom challenged me to be better with insight that he gained from over five decades of real-life experience coupled with an academic knowledge above many with Ph.D.s.

Chris Ganter, a friend and professional triathlete with a running background, also assisted me with what at one time was my Achilles heel: running. Just as I was starting to believe in my running, he gave me the support to know my running and be the runner.

Philippe Corre coached me while living in France and met me while embarking on a new chapter in life. Having just retired from being a professional triathlete, he fed me with a mutual love for running that kept my passion and drive alive. Many of the epiphanies and downloads for writing this book came while doing Philippe's workouts along the Northwest coast of France.

And thank you to the many students and athletes that I was fortunate to coach; you coached me in return. The experience from working with each one of you is invaluable, and the accumulation helps me evolve my understanding to aid the next relationship I'm fortunate to share a path with.

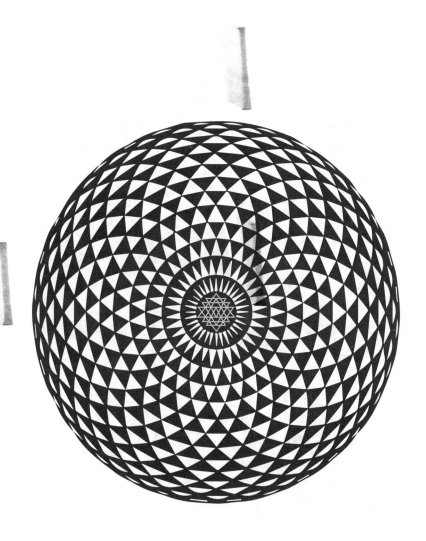

1
A BEGINNER'S
MIND

Part of the code to the art in *The Heart of Running* is tapping into what many consider the elusive *Runner's High*. This book will look to show you the paths to having a Runner's High each time you run. It is simple. That is not to say it is easy, but everyone with practice can achieve this flow in their running. With the right focus and knowing some paths to discovering these flow states, where you feel your best and perform your best, you too can activate your wings and fly when you run.

There is a short scene at the beginning of each chapter that illuminates some of the best "cards to play" for achieving a Runner's High. By paying attention to what is happening in these moments, you will have a glimpse and an understanding of the simple aspects of setting the stage for a Runner's High.

In this first scene, the runner is aware of the five senses. The internal dialogue between the body and mind is open and honest. The breath is a centerpiece to having the focus and the awareness of the moment. A deep compassion for the moment arises. A deep compassion for yourself arises. This compassion allows you to be the runner. This compassion allows you to tune in.

Fall in love with your running and, in the process, something much greater can happen. You can gain a compassionate life, a life you love.

SUNSET RUN

Imagine, with your heart, a beautiful runner. A graceful, efficient, and powerful runner. Imagine that runner is you. Running on a narrow dirt path, your eyes take in the horizon with only a peripheral awareness of ground beneath you. Your hips are hovering in balance with the earth below, the body straight, and the sky above. There is an awareness in the hips, a fulcrum and control center to your action. You know it well. The sound of your breath is pleasing. It hypnotizes you as it flows in and out, through you, around you. The breath is deep and fluid. Each expansion of the belly pulls in energy, fresh, bountiful energy. The easing of the diaphragm exhales the air back to the world precisely with a foot strike to the earth.

You are in sync now. You are dancing to a rhythm. Another foot strike and exhale, you hear it and feel it like the beating of a drum. Not just you, but the earth below, the sky above, and in you a deep-down yearning is quenched. You are resonating joy.

There is an orchestra within, merging with earth and sky. The rhythmic breathing is a wonder. The heart beats, the feet strike, and your spirit soars. Not only do you feel the earth, you smell the earth. The air has an ambiance to it; the colors give off emotions; the scents fill you with life. You have timed it perfectly, as the transition of the day to night is being displayed with a warm glow of colors and soft light on your skin. The light kindles a burning fire within. The love in the air is porous. At times you feel like crying at the awe of it all, but this morphs into an inner grin and an outer pace.

The pace is exhilarating. It is effortless. You are alive. You are alert. You are aware of everything. Everything you are doing in this amazing dance we call running is flawless. You become the runner. All this movement, all this effort, and yet you are still. You are as calm as you have ever been. You are at peace. You are the runner. You run on. On and on, mile after mile, strike after strike, breath after breath, chasing the setting sun.

FALL IN LOVE WITH RUNNING

You started off loving running. Go back to that first moment, those early childhood steps, those first running steps. You took them with a glimmer and radiance about you. Imagine your first running steps. Hopefully, one of your guardians was there to witness your beaming smile with a glow and sparkle in your eye. You feel the awe and the wonder of this controlled falling. You aren't entirely sure how long you can keep it up or how fast you can go, but you enjoy the fun. You are teetering on a disastrous fall at high speeds but somehow catch yourself with a quick footfall to the ground and another and another. "Hey," you think, "I've got this balance thing figured out," and bam, you tumble to the ground. It hardly phases you as you jump back to your feet and try this free-falling again and again. It is the time of your life. You are completely absorbed in this new discovery. The whole world melts away as you play with the form, with the steps, with the balance, with the timing of your first day running. It's a beautiful thing to have a beginner's mind.

"*I have just three things to teach: simplicity, patience, compassion. These three are your greatest treasures.*"

—Lao Tzu

The fortunate ones have not lost touch with their beginner mind. A choice and an approach to all of life's actions with the awe and splendor of growing and challenging and discovering something new. It is possible to go for your 10,001st run and marvel at the wonder and newness of it. To open a new door, run through it, and explore. There is always another door.

Every human should experience a vivid sunset run. If you are adept enough to experience a Runner's High (one path of thousands to a higher state of Being), day transitions are a playful time to go. Starting or finishing a run with a sunset is a way to set the "stage" and amplify the air, or actually, tap into the energy waiting for you to acknowledge it. Know this experience, and you will be motivated to know the sun's schedule and mirror it with yours—experiencing as many sunrises and sunsets as you can.

Maybe, if you were fully engaged in reading the first story about having a Pure Experience during the sunset run, if you gave your imagination its full attention and had no distractions, if you gave yourself fully to the task of "reading," maybe you entered into a bit of the Runner's High too? It is possible. A Runner's High has been verified by science and is not limited to running. Science calls it "flow" or being in a state of flow. But humans knew about flow long before science came along to measure it.

KNOWING YOUR TRUE ESSENCE

The heart of running is about awareness. The Japanese have a term for the highest level of awareness: Satori. Satori can be viewed a number of ways, one of which is to know the true essence. Satori is a comprehension and an understanding. While this teaching is about knowing your run, it is, on a deeper level, about discovering yourself and eventually knowing yourself. A master runner, or a

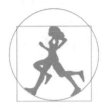

The fortunate ones have not lost touch with their **beginner mind**. A choice and an approach to all of life's actions with the awe and splendor of growing and challenging and discovering something new.

master of any craft, has a beautiful relationship with the body. He knows that the body's purpose is to serve the mind. The body can be viewed like a puppy, in that it is a curious, rambunctious, and lovable ball of energy that lives to be with and serve its master. It will do everything in its understanding and its will to please the master.

The mind and body relationship is crucial for a runner to thrive. The communication will need to be open and honest. Like any strong relationship, your body and mind will need to be born of truth and purpose. It is a mentor and apprentice connection. Unfortunately, for many in our society, the body is the mentor. While the body is a great and wonderful vehicle, it pales in comparison to the mind. For this affiliation to be fruitful, the mind cannot serve the body. The correct hierarchy, instead, is for the body to serve the mind. A runner explores this relationship and, while there is some trial and error, some in-fighting, some mistrust at times, and some blaming, in the end, the lessons only strengthen the bond.

But to know yourself, to awaken the runner within, you will need to adhere to another relationship within. The body is action and serves the mind; the mind is thinking and serves the soul. The soul knows. This is you. You are complex. Your Being is a body, mind, and soul. And the interactions, the relationships, are the inner workings of You. In order to feel and perform your best, you will have to know your running. To know your running, you will have to know yourself. *The Heart of Running* is about knowing your run and tasting the potential you will have to take part in the grandest journey of being human...discovering your Self.

The journey is life long and the paths you will discover are numerous.

Running is basic, primal, and an innate act to all the bipedal organisms. But how would humans match up to the other runners of the universe? How do humans match up on earth, compared to the animal kingdom?

Your first instinct might be to think, "Not that well." And you would be correct in a sense. After all, if you walk around New York City, you don't see a lot of humans ready to go toe-to-toe with a horse. And it's true. Even the fastest among us, Usain Bolt, cannot win a 100-meter dash against a cat. That's right, your lazy house cat would blow the socks off Bolt. We do not excel at short distance or sprinting events when compared to the animal kingdom. To say we don't excel might be a little gentle. In fact, we are pathetic when it comes to sprinting against animals. As athletes in general, even our strongest and fastest are weak and slow compared to other animals of our planet.

That's okay. We have to know our place in the world when it comes to physical abilities. In general, humans don't fair very well as compared to animals in physical abilities, but we do have one trait unmatched on earth: endurance. We are the endurance kings of the universe! Well, er, at least we are the endurance kings of earth!

The longer the run, the better humans perform against animals. Throw a little heat into the equation, and humans don't just outperform the rest of the animal kingdom, they far exceed it. At a certain point and distance, humans are the dominate endurance animals on earth. This is amazing, given the fact that every other measurable physical skill with human strength, speed, and the five senses are mediocre at best, and in the bottom half when compared to all the animals of earth. Yet humans reign supreme when it comes to endurance. This says a lot about you. Yes, you. Even if you haven't run very much, you are capable. Your very being here is a testament to your ancestors' abilities to run. To run for their lives! They ran for their lives (both metaphorically speaking and for real). That is why you can and should run for your life (both metaphorically speaking and maybe for real).

Matter of fact, humans are so good at endurance running that it has become one of those quintessential traits, like our big brain and tool-making abilities that science equates with the evolution of our species. It may even be the catalyst for our big brains and tool-making abilities!

Humans are not just *better* at endurance; they are far superior. Man's ability to cool himself while running makes him about the only species effective at covering distance in the heat of the day. Humans are able to do what is called *persistence hunting*, where they run and track down their prey to exhaustion. Antelope, deer, even the fastest animal on earth, a cheetah, will succumb to our superior endurance.

What you should realize here is that humans have this incredible ability—the potential to outrun the world. This says a lot about you. Think about it. Not just in terms of running but in terms of the potential to have physical stamina outlasting the entire animal kingdom. Humans persevere and, in fact, can thrive when others suffer. This is a talent innate in humans. A talent innate in you.

ENDURANCE IS WITH YOU. WHERE ARE YOU?

Endurance is inside of you—part of you—even though many are not aware of their endurance. It takes practice—daily practice—to bring it out. It takes concentration and focus. It takes determination and patience. It means being dedicated to yourself through relationships. It takes...okay, wait for it, this is a bad word to many of you...exercise. If it is not a bad word to you, then you already have discovered a big secret. Because for those of you who are aware of your gifts, *exercise* is just a term used to describe your empowered play.

While this teaching is about knowing your running, the superior endurance of humans can manifest itself in a number of other endurance activities. Any activity that will sustain your effort and a deeper rhythmic breathing can be a display of human endurance. Dancing, swimming, hockey...to rattle off a few.

You know how good exercise is for you—it is marketed everywhere and by many experts. You are told how important it is...how you can prevent this and get that. You know exercise is good for you, but why do so many dislike it? Especially when endurance is a "human trait."

To add a layer to this, we know the recipe for having your health span and your life span match:

Your prescription:
Six days a week for the rest of your life: ~~exercise~~
PLAY.

Some of you will throw your hands to the sky, jump up and down, and yell, "Yes!" Some of you will throw your hands to the sky, jump up and down, and...cry. If you are crying, you are still stuck on the exercise bit. There are foot strikes to take and paths to follow that are attractive and fun when applied from the knowledge of knowing your next best step. For those of you who are excited, there will be paths to take again with fresh eyes, there will be new paths, there will be mysterious paths. All these paths will lead you on a journey to self-discovery, self-improvement, and faster, more enjoyable running.

Like any skill or talent, like any God-given gift, you will need to water the desert flower for it to flourish. For those of you aware of your gifts and for those who appreciate them, practice is not so much about training as it is about something much more. It becomes an expression, a form of communication, a way to realize your potential, a way to engage in meaningful relationships. It is *empowering yourself to play*. If you apply your gifts with true purpose, if you can be intrinsically motivated about your abilities, if you achieve balance in your life, then training your talents should feel much less like work and much more like play.

From here on out, consider yourself fortunate when you go for a run; be thankful for the time; be grateful for the environment; be appreciative of the vigor to want to run. This is a first step—a big and powerful step—for empowering yourself to play and achieving a Runner's High each time you put on your running shorts.

Empowering yourself to play is a major attitude shift for most when it comes to exercise. You can do this alone or amplify the playing effect with others. Play is right alongside endurance as one of those quintessential human traits. To be able to "practice" your gifts daily, to be able to explore the depths of your talent, you will need to play. This is the natural and sustainable way. You've gotta play!

"Play is the highest form of research."

—Albert Einstein

2
REASONS FOR
RUNNING

Consider the Runner's High as a survival mechanism. Our ancestors used the flow states that we refer to as the Runner's High to stay alive. The raw aspect of running in the wilderness in search of food is an element that forces the present moment on you. Being in the present moment is a requirement for finding a flow state. The Runner's High is a simple matter of paying attention. But this paying attention is not easy. It takes mindful practice to achieve.

THE HUNT

Sky Eagle's heart beats stronger in anticipation of the hunt. His tribe finished the last of the winter rations about seven days ago. The weather finally has warmed the earth enough that Sky Eagle will lead his warriors on the first hunt in many weeks. A word is not spoken as the hunting party gathers at the edge of camp, and together, as one, they all begin running.

The party is made up of men, women, and children old enough to begin learning the ways of the hunt. All play a crucial and equal role supporting each other; the mentoring process is seamless, invisible.

For a moment their minds wonder. This simple pleasure of embarking on a hunt on foot invigorates the spirit. They move swiftly, silently, like owls gliding in the air. The life force spikes in each of them as they climb and climb up the side of a mountain. Breathing well while ascending a mountain pumps the brain with endorphins as blood flows vigorously through the body. Getting out of camp and covering some ground give their focus a precision. It is there that a transformation takes place. Their senses are on alert. Something basic takes over as the tribe is able to run for the thrill but also with a sense of urgency as their families back home are becoming hungry.

The hunting expedition is capable of covering vast amounts of land in search of prey. Running Bear is concerned for his wife and newborn daughter, knowing they are hungry and counting on him to find something to eat. Crazy Horse is the first to see them—a large buck and several does. She motions to the party, and instinctively the strategy is set. As they are running east, into the wind, Crazy Horse covers the perimeter from the south, Running Bear covers the perimeter from the north, and Sky Eagle leads the remainder through the middle. The party braces for what could go on all day, even into the night and the next day. Each movement calculated and efficient. Not a single breath wasted. This will take everything they are capable of—and maybe more.

They chase the herd deeper and deeper into the mountains. They run up and down ridges, over saddles, across creeks and rivers, slowly depleting the herd's ability to continue. They have been running all through the night and are anticipating the dawn as the end of night brings a stillness to the air.

Running Bear smells the air and picks up sage brush, decomposing leaves, mud from melting snow puddles, and...a hint of the exhausted prey he has been hunting all night. Scanning the hillside, he notices movement up on a craggy outcropping. One of the does is hiding under some trees in a last, desperate attempt to avoid the hunters. Adrenalin spikes through Running Bear's system as his body moves with stealth and efficiency. In one fluid motion, the spear raises above his head with his elbow pointing right at the target. The speed of the attack startles the deer, and it hesitates for an instant. It bounds up the hill, but it's already too late. The thrust of Running Bear's arrow rock meets the flesh of the deer's neck. It is a decisive blow. The tribe will feast tonight.

YOU WERE BORN TO RUN

You can all run. You have this gift. This is part of being human—our stunning ability for endurance running. You are built from the ground up to run! Humans are the physical specimens for but one skill on this planet: endurance running. Let's celebrate our greatness!

But where are all the runners? Sure, marathons are booming and you see runners at the park, but really, where are all the runners? According to runningusa.org, 19 million runners finished running events in 2013. That's a lot of runners, right? While not all runners are going to race and compete, that still leaves 300 million or 99.5 percent of the population who did not take part in an organized group run.

So, if humans are so natural at running, so gifted at it, why aren't more of us running? Because the approach and reasons to do so are off balance. Many are taking their ability for granted, rarely paying attention to the form and the movement. Many are just "doing" running, and it's a mechanical approach. The trick is to bio-hack and upgrade your running with awareness. To take it up a notch by connecting the heart and mind awareness. Again, it is simple with profound implications, but simple does not equate to easy. When you love to run and have a focused and relaxed mind, the heart and mind can take your abilities to another level. But many run with little awareness, allowing the autonomic nervous system to take charge by default so that the brain can think about what's for dinner. Or they run to listen to music or to solve a problem. This is a mistake. When you are running, simply run, with your whole body (body, mind, heart, and soul).

Society has lost touch with the correct reasons to run. Many are not tapping into the tribe and the relationships that take running to the next level. (Because those who do run are often running with little attention.) Many of you are running mechanically. Many are slaves to the numbers. Most of you are running to get something in return. Many of you are distracted from your action. Many running role models go too hard or too long or too much without enough balance. And, for too many, the mind rules over the body like a slave: "Shut up legs and go faster." For the very unfortunate, the body is ruling the mind, where body image is king. For many, a Runner's High is fleeting and elusive and very difficult to attain.

If you run to look good, lose weight, be fast, eat whatever you want, be healthy, or avoid disease, then you are missing a major opportunity. You are squandering your gift. While these are all benefits to running, they are unfortunate reasons for running.

If you run with the mindset of getting something out of it, if you run because you know it makes you healthy, you are missing the point. While it is better to run than not to—no matter your motivation—running for the right reason, you will find, is so much more rewarding. Why do you run? Or perhaps, why don't you run?

If you run for the right reasons, not only do you still get all the benefits of running, but you do so in a balanced and sustainable way. If you run to lose weight, what happens when you lose the weight? Do you keep on running? Maybe, maybe not. When you run to look good, how much does running feel like work? How much fun is it when you are running to get something in return?

The answers will vary, and to be fair, you can derive a good deal of fun out of running even if you are only doing it so you can eat anything and everything you want and still keep an athletic body.

But you can tap into a deeper level; you can enjoy your running even more if you do it for one simple reason…you love running! That's it. Those other things are benefits of running, and while you like those benefits, they should not be your reason for running. Otherwise, you won't reach your potential, you won't sustain your running, and you won't enjoy it to its full capacity.

To begin a journey of loving your running takes a simple action: you must pay attention. Running with heart and feeling the love are about being aware. Awareness. This is simple but something you can spend a lifetime growing. The result of expanding your awareness is more joy. That's where looking at any exercise that you do as empowered play can elevate your abilities. Playing is a high level of engagement, and you seek out and perform play just to play. Not for any external reward if you are truly in the element and playing. This is you beginning to understand how to thrive not just in running but in any action.

When kids play, consider the relationships they create both internally and externally. Lifelong friends are born from play. Paths are forged for understanding what drives purpose and meaning from play. Play is growing and evolving into a better person. Play is understanding how to interact with different

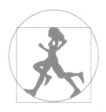

If you run to look good, lose weight,

be fast, eat whatever you want, be

healthy, or avoid disease, then **you are**

missing a major opportunity. You are

squandering your gift.

people. Play will test your boundaries and help you break through into new realms. Play is the fastest way to forge relationships in powerful, meaningful ways. For the best runners, running is play.

You can all run. Just like dolphins swim, humans run. We are these marvelous endurance runners. You are an endurance runner in your core, in your heart. However, life in today's society is killing running. Running is being attacked from every angle. Even many well-intentioned running experts are inadvertently throwing water on the fire. Making running about the myriad of external benefits you can obtain, rather than the simple joy of the action itself. Instead, a goal should be about the powerful life-changing relationships you can build from running. The deep and profound yearning to be connected can be as simple as going for a run with a friend. You may communicate directly or indirectly, but either way, it is powerful to run with someone in silence or to ponder some of life's questions. The shared experience will be meaningful.

BE A MOVER, A RUNNER

A child growing up in today's world might rightly state that dolphins swim and humans sit. The research on sitting is dire. You would rather smoke a pack of cigarettes by lunchtime than sit for eight hours every day. In terms of your health, in your ability to live, the smoker will statistically outlast the sitter. Sitting is corroding humans from the inside out. Sitting is dulling our body, our mind, and our spirit, and society continues to turn a blind eye to what humans are. Part of the essence of being human is being a runner. Certainly, being a mover, a thing of action, a human being, not a human sitting.

To that point many are human doings. Everyone is busy *doing*. Just doing a run is missing the opportunity of *being* a runner. Be the runner. "BeRun!" Blur the boundaries between you and the action of running into one. Merge into the form of the runner, the whole-body runner.

You have this innate gift, this package someone carefully wrapped and wants you to open. Many never open the package, disliking the wrapping. And, understandably so, given how running is marketed, taught, perceived, and done by most in society. Others open up the package, try it on, and quickly toss it aside thinking, "It doesn't fit me." Many of you get distracted and take the path society has paved, and guess what, it's all downhill. (Metaphorically, the bells and whistles are selling you distractions and shortcuts. There are no shortcuts, and running well means no distractions.) Part of the problem is the ease for humans to initiate a running program with little or no experience and support.

From top to bottom, it is easy to walk out your front door and go for a run. This can be the crux of the matter—but also its beauty. You go for a run and assume you are doing it right. Never considering the flaw in your approach. You progress a number of weeks, months even, because humans are awesome at running. You develop a few less-than-ideal habits, like foot striking before your plumb line. The plumb line being a weighted string that you could hypothetically hang from your center to the ground. A root cause from a combination of weak glutes, poor balance, pelvic tilt, and plantar flexion of the foot. All pretty easy problems to fix, but much, much harder to unlearn.

The greater impact from your poor form is manifesting stress in a number of places, namely your foot, ankles, and knees, but sometimes with the wrong impact, it shoots into your femur, heading into your hips and lower back. Your body is healthy, you are running smart, eating right, sleeping well, but as your running program progresses, you begin to have some niggles and wiggles. Some of the foot and ankle pains force you to skip a run or two here and there, but you do not think much of it. Then, out of nowhere, shin splints. You ignore them at first, but after a quick run on a hard surface, the shin splints become a little more than just bothersome. You take a week off from running. You question your body. You question your will power. You question your shoes. You question your program. You question your supporters. But mostly, you question yourself. Maybe running is just not for you? There is one question you forgot to ask. One question you did not take a deeper look into. By considering it, you can get to the root of your problem.

You forgot to question your form and your overall approach to running. You considered it for a second: "It's not perfect, but it's pretty good, right?" You consider your form good enough and move along to the next grief counselor, your shoes. "It's gotta be the shoes. Not enough support. Or too much heel drop. Maybe not enough arch support? I should buy this shoe since its increased technology says it will lower the impact. Or maybe this minimalist approach will correct my foot strike. Perfect! Problem solved. Who's ready to run!?"

If you are not a beginner runner and are moderately advanced or advanced, the crux is often a strong focus on fitness and strength, as opposed to form and grace. Many of the more advanced runners are slaves to the numbers. They consider themselves "runners," they like it and even love it, but they are running mechanically. They are mostly concerned with getting faster, stronger, going longer, and focusing on a narrow band of running: fitness. They are running "doers" and not running Beings.

Being a slave to the numbers also means being a slave to the technology. The issue is using the technology from the realm of a thinking and calculating brain. You are bombarded with constant distractions meant to "tune" you into running. What is your heart rate, your pace, how far you have gone, and how much farther do you have to go, mixed in with beeps and, most likely, some music. All distractions from your true relationship with running. How can you connect to your inner knowing with so much external information? With each distraction, the brain is activated, taking away the potential for stillness.

BE FOCUSED, NOT DISTRACTED

Stillness is the most powerful use of the running mind. The surface of this mind is like that of a perfectly reflective mountain lake. Being a slave to the technologies is like backing up a dump truck and unloading a ton of stones to send ripples across the surface. Noise. Distraction from the true beauty before you and in you.

So use the technology and use the numbers, but do not be a slave to them. Understanding whether the information is a distraction—or a focus—is an important question. Do not confuse a stimulation with focus. Often, this outside information is stimulating the brain and/or body in such a way as to rule out the soul from entering the playground.

Technology can assist with dialing in biofeedback as well as communicating with a coach—both important aspects of evolving your knowledge of running. But the deepest form of biofeedback is being in touch with your body/mind/soul complex. There is no better way to match up your top-end form with your top-end fitness and know the right pace, instant to instant, than to know your form.

You are seeking balance and harmony within so that a deep awareness, a timeless appreciation for each pixel of your movement, can be known. For many, it is easy to stimulate the body and the mind. How do you stimulate the soul? Harmony.

Harmony is with You. Where are You?

With an active and engaged neutrality to the body and brain, the soul can be heard and felt. This portal is through the heart. The joy of the soul participating in life is beyond any feeling the mind might conjure on its own. This is the recipe for creating your running talent. Do you understand the depth of running with heart?

The point is to seek harmony in your approach to running. With an open heart and a beginner's mind, achieve instant balance with your Being and your action. Give yourself completely to the task. With an awareness that cuts across the spectrum, you can know fitness and form on intimate levels. Love and respect each component and appreciate the relationship that you have with your form and your fitness. The two are woven together, and both will need your heartfelt attention to thrive in running. You must feel the interconnectedness to know it. The joy of a Pure Experience happens at the point where your form and fitness match up on a moment-by-moment basis, while in complete awareness. You can only achieve this with your full and absolute attention. It will take practice. If you are on the right path, the practice is the reward.

Watch kids running, and you will see how "it" is done on many levels. Not only do children run simply because it is fun, they run with ease and balance. To a trained eye, the foot strike and balance match any track star. Unless you were a fortunate child to consistently run into adulthood and enjoy the process with knowledgeable coaching and intrinsic motivation, your form and balance will need focus. It's a lot like learning a second language. If you learn at a young age and continue learning the language, you have no accent and are articulate like a native. If you learn as an adult, you will have an accent and have distinct signs (flaws) from your first language. Of course, you can obtain the native tongue, but it takes a lot of practice.

If you were an adult learning how to swim for the first time, support and mentoring would be essential. Although running may be more natural for humans, it still takes mentoring and/or high levels of awareness to get it right. You can learn on your own, but not without impressive amounts of study. Having a mentor will speed your journey along and increase your capacity to pause, reflect, and share the insight with another.

YOUR RUNNING MENTOR

Running will thrive (let's say 10 percent of the population actively enjoys running instead of less than 1 percent) when there is a system of mentors and apprentices that branch off into a web where everyone is both a mentor and apprentice with another, including all ages and abilities for the whole of society. Imagine all the people living in harmony. It is easy if you build tribes in the modern world, tribes with the purpose of having fun with play and interactions to discover a deeper meaning and yearning for all.

Imagine a society where there is a continuum of running, where kids who love to run (all kids given the opportunity with the correct approach) continue running. Running for the right reason. Running because they love to run. It is so human to run. What if society instilled a value of running, not born of health, not born of winning the race, not born of avoiding dis-ease, but born of fun? What if running focused on play? Play with as many relationships as possible. Running in all its wondrous forms. What a fun dream!

Imagine the dismay of our ancestors who loved to run, now seeing how we live our lives. To run for fun, to run simply because you can, not because you are hungry and surviving. But that is not what happened. Not by a long shot. Our ancestors are laughing at us. "Silly people, trying to be something they are not."

Too many people have lost touch with the running equation as it relates to one of their innate gifts. They look in a mirror full of lights and colors and distractions, not noticing the endurance animal, not looking into its eyes. Is a dolphin ever going to find happiness if you take away its ability or desire to swim? It is a pretty clear answer. So, why do humans think they can find happiness by avoiding one of their basic gifts?

Instead of taking the bait for a marketing ad and some reward for running, be intrinsically motivated. There is a paradox to being intrinsically versus externally motivated. Intrinsic motivation carries a lot more passion, a lot more depth, a lot more strength than external motivation. All benefits you obtain from running are an effect that you may or may not receive as external rewards. Research from the 70s will highlight this over-justification effect that happens when your motivation for a given action is externally rewarded.

Greene, Sternberg, and Lepper (1976) played mathematical games with schoolchildren, which the children seemed to enjoy. After a while, they started giving rewards for success. When they took away the rewards, the children quickly gave up playing the games.

The explanation was that the children had decided that they were playing for the reward, not for the fun.

So, why do you run? You run because it is fun. That's it. You literally enjoy the action of running. By approaching your running this way, not only do you obtain all its benefits, but you achieve them with deeper satisfaction and understanding. Secondly, you open up the doors for reaching your true capacity with running.

But there is another good answer. If you run to improve your relationships both within yourself and with others, then you are on the right track. However, the path that will branch off like an old oak tree in a meadow is a general sense of play while running.

YOUR RUNNING, YOUR PASSION

There are many doors that open while running with intrinsic motivation, doors that lead to other doors. Unfortunately, many runners don't have the key. One of the important doors to open, now that you have the intrinsic motivation key, is the Passion Door. You already have opened up the biggest, most impressive door, the Fun Door, which allowed you to open a vast realm, but first you peek to see what lies behind this door of passion.

Passion allows you to have curiosity, still more doors, and the combination of fun + passion + curiosity, while running means that you discover. What do you discover? How to run really well. Sounds pretty simple, right? It is, but the path is long, and it will help you a great deal to have support along the way. You can do it alone, but it takes much longer and the satisfaction is dulled. This is really just a way to break up the essence of play into smaller parts. What is fun, passion, and curiousness but play itself. While it is possible to play well by yourself, the potential amplification effect with others is fantastic.

Too much fun + passion + curiosity can lead to ambition. This is where some patience will help you balance out the equation. Your body and mind can only absorb so much. It is easy for the mind to get well ahead of the body. This goes back to building a relationship with purpose and honesty. You will have to listen to your body. Your body will tell you what a sustainable pace for progress is, but you will need to be mindful to its subtle and not so subtle communication.

You see, another key aspect to running is the relationships. The relationships within yourself between your body, mind, and soul and also the relationships with others. When two people, both intrinsically motivated, team up for a task (this could be two in close balance or apprentice and mentor), they are both now capable of achieving so much more.

The power of a positive relationship, a relationship born of purpose and based on truth, is electric, and the force is strong. Not just in the fun you will have, but in your understanding of who you are—one of the greatest gifts a person can have.

To summarize the teaching to this point, the aim of *The Heart of Running* is to know your running. In order to do this, you must have a purposeful and honest relationship with yourself, which then allows you to have the same with others. You will have to know and understand the hierarchy of the soul, mind, and body and be motivated to know yourself through intrinsic motivation, which is really about playing and building relationships. Running well is simply about awareness. Lastly, the teaching has conveyed that you have a gift for endurance.

Endurance is with You. Where are You?

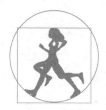

The power of a positive relationship, a relationship born of purpose and based on truth, is electric, and the force is strong. Not just in the fun you will have, but **in your understanding of who you are**—one of the greatest gifts a person can have.

3
COACHING
AS PLAY

What is play at the highest order, but a state of flow, a Runner's High. How do you describe play? What are the key elements? What in your daily life are you doing to drop into a play state? Kids have a natural tendency to play—we all do—but many of us lose touch with it as we "mature." A crucial element to the art in the heart of running is to play. Empower yourself to play. Running is one of a million different ways to play.

Playing is about paying attention and challenging your abilities. When your activities become about empowered play, you begin tapping into your potential.

TRUE PLAY IS
MINDFULNESS

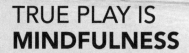

"Play is the beginning of knowledge."

—George Dorsey

Standing in a park, you observe your three-year-old boy chasing your five-year-old daughter in a loose game of "cat and mouse" or "catch me if you can." Both are engaged in an ancient game that has been playing out for eons. At its core, the game is simply the thrill of running. The contrast between the hunter and the hunted. Both kids are boisterous and clearly in a state of joy. The imaginations of the greater implications of the game manifest with fast feet and wide smiles.

They challenge each other in a sort of dance as both brush up against their current abilities and push beyond naturally. The instinctual play is teaching this brother and sister so much about relationships. You see this simple game addressing physical, emotional, cognitive, social, and moral development. The glue that ties it all together and fosters growth is laughter. The drama unfolding before you is the essence of humankind's highest display of intelligence. In your stillness, you hear that inner child begging to participate in the play. You ease into the game, utilizing all life's experience to elevate the play to its highest order. Laughter is the ultimate prize.

LEARN BY TEACHING

A great teacher knows how to produce the passion spark and ignite the heart's gift.

It has been said, "To master something, first you must teach it." In becoming a coach or teacher you are honoring The Way (the creation of mentors teaching mentors to pass along and share knowledge for the betterment of all) by serving others and sparking curiosity to open new doors and explore. You are passing along the gifts that you have earned from the experience of your relationships. While engaging with the kids you are coaching (or anyone), you become aware of insight, new insight that somehow escaped you all these years while you practiced running. Who is teaching who, you wonder?

The preferred way for humans to learn about their world is through play. The inner child in you is asking to play right now. At the heart of each of you is an inner presence ready to explore, willing and asking to play daily. This chapter will focus on the best practices for teaching running to children, but uses your imagination to expand this into the world of adult running too. If you can obtain a beginner mind like a child does, be intrinsically motivated, and play with your running "focus," then you are realizing your moment in its fullest.

"The superior teacher demonstrates, the great teacher inspires."

—William Arthur Ward

Teaching children to run does not take an expert in running as much as it takes an expert in being human. The core of your teaching should come from your heart, using running as a tool to directly and indirectly express greater life lessons.

It is the view of this teaching that *play* is the highest level of awareness for learning anything. The gift of running, at its core and its essence, is a playful nature. If you can shift your view of running from work or exercise and know it for what it is truly meant to be, play, then you will take paths with the most potential for growth. You take these paths with a mindset deserving of all the splendor and awe they encourage. Each moment a teachable experience in the awareness of play.

As stated earlier, the quality of your experience with any action is dependent on the motivation. For the highest quality experience, something also known as Pure Experience, and simply, play, it is important that you find the action inherently interesting and enjoyable because you are intrinsically excited. In other words, you are personally choosing the activity as a means for growth and self-discovery. If, like many, you are performing an action for a dissociated outcome or an external reward, then the entire action will be dulled. Do not run for health reasons, money, social status, or any other external reward. You can like these benefits, but do not confuse them with your reason for running. Play is the ultimate form of growth and self-discovery. The qualities derived from play are the best reasons for running.

This is your bridge for reaching out to kids and teaching them the lessons of being a better *runner*. What an impactful way to serve others and make a difference all in the name of play—fostering a space for kids to nurture growth through play, establishing challenges and lessons that gain the most participation, creating meaningful relationships, and assisting with a child's teaching and learning process—these are at the heart of teaching children.

Play is a simple concept that has a depth that makes it hard both to define or to master. Recognize the beauty in these simple concepts—life is full of them. Becoming a student of these simple concepts and utilizing a beginner mind each time you step on the path is an unlimited source of growth. With a beginner's mind, you may discover something new with each run. Some essential qualities to play are as follows: autonomy, freedom, expression, curiosity, exploration, personally directed role playing, imagination, connection, spontaneous creativity, and challenging actions to practice with a general sense of fun that incorporates laughter, often in a space that facilitates a shared experience for relationship development. The best coaches in the world are the ones who have an ability to connect, facilitate, and support an environment conducive for play.

Coaches working with children have a wonderful opportunity for growth. The teaching/learning and learning/teaching loop with children is multifaceted. Being a mentor of children is a sacred honor and the teaching in not one directional. As much as you might instill and facilitate knowledge (through play if you are an expert), your apprentices (the kids are the true masters of play) will be teaching you just as much. The best coaches are learning something with each and every relationship while teaching. In this way both are expanding their awareness. If you want to learn how to run well faster, try teaching it.

FACILITATING PLAY

Your first objective as a coach for children is to be a facilitator of play. With practice and training, you will realize the journey is endless. To be a facilitator of play means you cannot be too controlling, there cannot be too many rules, you cannot put too much pressure on outcome, and you cannot provide too many rewards. You will need to be supportive and fair and seek out participation. You will need to celebrate the process and take each instant as a teachable moment without always intervening. Children learn through experience, with trial and error. Allowing them to fail and experience the sliding scale of error is key. With repetition and practice, they will learn the tricks to becoming more proficient. In many ways, the more they fail, through the attitude of play, the more experience they have and therefore the more apt they become. Eventually, a breakthrough will open the door for the next level of play and will yield everlasting breakthroughs in improving abilities. Set up an environment where the kids feel safe failing. Recognize the learning process involved in failing. Celebrate the growth and encourage this self-discovery.

Allow the kids to be the driver of their personal play and its characteristics. But be supportive and encouraging from a standpoint of recognizing their path. A good coach will observe the nuances of each child's play and have an intuitive sense for their personal next best step in development. This is not limited to their next step in running but their next step in life; an expert coach knows the two are linked.

By setting the stage for play, you are optimizing a critical element for evolution in life: relationship building. What better way to know your peers, interact, and grow than to play? As a coach, getting all the kids to interact as richly as possible, and for each to recognize the value in every team member, will take everyone's play to the next level. An expert coach will blur the lines between the stereotypes and allow teamwork to take place on a level of unity sought after by all. Unleash the power of the group dynamics and the potential for each peer to be a teacher. Let the strong support the weak in a process that makes both stronger. If you want to build character, build a sense of connection between each team member. The most powerful connections are often the ones that on the surface don't seem to fit.

The Way is simple. Mentors support apprentices who mentor others in an ongoing process that creates relationships for growth and understanding at each level. Service to others is one of your highest purposes. See the dynamic qualities here: By being a good student, you are servicing a mentor, and by being a good mentor, you are servicing a student. Finding the activity and the relationship that will resonate with you will give you a deep sense of meaning, feelings of being connected, and set you on a path to fulfilling your purpose. And so goes *the* Way.

A wonderful aspect of play is its ability to spark, cultivate, and grow a relationship. Relationships both internally with your body, mind, and soul and also with others, animals included. If you have been fortunate to run with a dog, you have witnessed the unfettered joy of playful running. While you are most likely the master to your dog, the dog is teaching you a valuable life lesson:

to give yourself fully to the task and run with all the pleasure showcased by your happy dog.

Beyond this: If you are in a position to coach children, be aware of your sacred opportunity. Start with a simple foundation of play so that you may spark, cultivate, and grow relationships. This is one of the highest duties you can perform. You evolve through relationships; you learn through relationships; you discover who you are through relationships. If you can enable relationships with meaning and purpose, consider yourself most fortunate. The relationships you create are the only thing you keep for your entire life. This importance cannot be overstated.

Running can be a catalyst for deeper relationship development both internally and externally. This is the gift.

Cherish your relationships. Teach and coach others to do the same.

Teaching our children? Hmm, sometimes this teaching/learning loop is one sided. What are we learning from our children? The masters of play. Too much adult teaching will indoctrinate them with all the rules, pressures, and successes of adult life. It's time to let our children be children; it's time to learn from them as much as we might try to teach them. If we become aware and allow them to drive their play and build relationships in the process, then we lay the groundwork for not just better runners but better human beings, the real goal of any youth activity.

"This is the real secret of life—to be completely engaged with what you are doing in the here and now. And instead of calling it work, realize it is play."

—Alan W. Watts

Youth sports for the vast majority of kids are in crisis. Society is infusing youth activities with characteristics of "adult" worries, aspirations, fears, successes, recognition, rewards, and security. Teaching a methodical approach, making many mechanical in their approach to seeking the rewards and recognition of the system. Instead, infuse youth activities with heart. Your heart. If you start from here, you will know what to do.

Focusing on the process and not the outcome will be an important step in the right direction. With the right process, the outcome will be a win-win situation. But children should hardly care if they themselves are winners. Children just want to participate and have fun. The process (PLAY) is the outcome, and it is the best teacher anyone can enlist. The hypercompetitive nature is not a healthy growth at any level and certainly a poison for children. This drive to be the best, fastest, strongest, and most elite is corroding the heart and soul of youth activities. Being your best goes way beyond winning. Unfortunately, many are stuck on this path toward evolution, assuming that this performance goal will bring all the feelings of deeper meaning and purpose we are all in search of. Yet winning and performing well will not bring fulfillment even if it brings all those external rewards like recognition, awards, and money.

Being competitive can be useful for growth only when it is applied from its true meaning. Today's understanding of competition has been skewed into *the activity or condition of striving to gain or win something by defeating or establishing superiority over others.* A Chinese proverb states, "The beginning of wisdom is to call things by their right name." The root meaning of competition is very different from what is commonly viewed today.

From late Latin, *competere,* "strive in common" in classical Latin means "to come together, agree, to be qualified, strive together;" from *com* "together" to *petere* "to strive and seek." Competition's root meaning and true meaning for growth is to strive together for the attainment of something. To go forth together to understand each other's potential. True competition is striving for excellence together. In this way, competition is an opportunity for enjoying a quest to achieve personal and perhaps team potential. The best effort of another has the potential to bring out the best effort in you. There are no winners and losers. Just an attempt to raise the level of play in a way that everyone benefits from a challenging learning experience.

You cannot let the hypercompetitive adult teaching of winning and being the best take center stage in any child's development. Children will naturally strive toward self-improvement given the support they need. If you want to see just how talented children are, facilitate true competition—to go forth together and naturally push abilities—with a sense that the "competitors" are your brothers and sisters enjoying the same skills you are fostering. Sharing, showing, and challenging each other to continue growing. If the foundation for this competition is layered in play for relationship development, then you are not only providing a wonderful service for the children but a wonderful service for your community.

With this type of foundation for teaching children, they will self-improve to levels unheard of today. They will do it with more character, and they will do it by lifting up the peers around them. It will come naturally because it is part of their personal self-development. The parents are there to observe and support, the coaches are there mostly for this, too, while much of the teaching comes from simply facilitating fair play and full participation so that they can trial and error their skill.

"If you want to be creative, stay in part a child, with the creativity and invention that characterizes children before they are deformed by adult society."

—Jean Piaget

You can see this play out time and time again with an activity like running. You start off loving running as an essential element for active play. If you go back far enough, maybe all the way back to those first running steps, you started off running with a smile on your face. Running is the critical act in many sports and, at first, hopefully, you engaged in running from a standpoint of true play. You did, if your mentors, coaches, and parents didn't turn the play into a "deformed adult society," where the pressure to perform with concrete rules and the seriousness of adult-like success poisoned the game.

Running in its true form is play. Society will quickly morph running into exercise for external reward. This blurs the beauty, the gift, and the power of running. To follow running paths to new heights and discover new paths, the core of your motivation comes from play. This is a central teaching in this book.

What is play but an expression of the heart?

In its true form, play and mindfulness become synonymous. The correlation in being connected, relaxed, aware, completely present, and in a state of bliss is clear to see. In this sense, play is a door, an opening, a path towards being mindful in every breath you take. Play is the highest order and action of mindfulness. The beauty and the gift are that this is natural. Watch children, even with a limited amount of support, given an opportunity, play will grow. It is a most resilient seed planted in each of you. Play. Just add water daily and see the plant flourish. Grow your play.

If you mentor children, do you facilitate—or control—play? Often adults want to be in complete authority and have every moment under control when they are teaching. It is important to be able to let go of some of this control. To organize a space, a game, establish some loose rules so that the children are the center of developing their play and expanding on the simple parameters given. They discover their creative potential in doing this. Sometimes the biggest role of a coach is keeping it fair by allowing for the greatest amount of participation.

Play has an element of chaos and freedom. The ability to be

creative and spontaneous. The motivation for play is internal and the only way to keep it eternal. It comes from within and is born of simple desires and is hard to force. Intrinsic motivation is key. This is a powerful force. This is a force with all the potential for all those great things we want to instill in our children but, with good intentions, often wind up taking shortcuts that lead into box canyons. For play to flourish and bring forth the passion, meaning, and purpose, the motivation must be intrinsic. This means children are driving and facilitating the action through simple aspects of curiosity and interest.

The best thing a coach or parent can do is to be supportive and to enjoy observing. Just being there to observe and be present in their play. One of the most powerful things you can say is that you enjoyed watching. That's it. It doesn't matter if they did "well" or "poorly," you simply enjoyed watching the process and were there to support their interests. The learning process can be accelerated when those tough experiences sink in, and the lesson is understood; at that moment you become stronger.

Knowing the true definition of competition—to go forth together and explore the possibilities of their abilities—you can begin to see some creative and insightful paths that children can take in their development.

FOSTER PLAY TO DEVELOP RELATIONSHIPS TO SPARK COMPETITION

This is the way to ignite a fierce passion for improvement through self-discovery. Running is but one potential catalyst.

What is play, flow, mindfulness, Runner's High...Pure Experience, but the highest achievement of humans? Here is the truth of the matter: all these mystical states are born of the heart. The heart and bringing forth the strongest emotion, the strongest energy in the universe. Resonating love. It is easy to do this with something you love, like running. The trick is understanding the action enough to apply to *any* action. As a coach who understands this principle, you can move mountains by supporting and amplifying each child you come in contact with. With kids, a portal is always play.

Play is with You. Where are You?

4
EATING WITH
HEARTFULNESS

Achieving your potential is about growing your ability to pay attention. Expanding your awareness is another way of being in flow states, another way of achieving your potential. While harmonizing the internal body, a vast universe with more cells than stars in the Milky Way galaxy, the whole body can act together as one heart beating to the rhythm of your action. A heart, mind, and body in sync and energizing your motion is a key discovery to transforming into an aware runner. A runner experiencing the Runner's High.

By aligning the heart, body, and mind with a focus on your motion, you move beyond the motion. You move into the strongest forces of your consciousness. This is the beginning of an alliance, a way of creating a bridge between your body, mind, and heart. By honoring this alliance, a deeper appreciation, a deeper love, is known. Here, you communicate to every cell in your body with one clear voice.

Intent is king. Your attitude, your belief, and what you know are very powerful tools. When you expand your awareness and put conscious intent into the food you eat, you are aligning a force that will shift your health and the way your body utilizes the energy from your food. You will begin to make decisions that affect not just what you eat, but more importantly, how you eat. Align your whole being, align the trillions of cells in your body, with one purpose—that you love the food you are eating and that you appreciate the nutrition it will bring your body.

What relationship do you have with your food? What vibration, what force, what intent are you sending to the food that enters your body? Are you showing up and truly paying attention and being grateful for the food that enters your temple?

Just like you learn to pay attention to a singular purpose while you run, learn to have a singular focus when you eat.

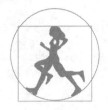

Align your **whole being**, align the trillions of cells in your body, with one purpose—that you love the food you are eating and that you **appreciate the nutrition** it will bring your body.

SENDING A BOOM, BOOM, BOOM

Looking out over the vast landscape, you see all. You feel the planet and the solar system revolving around the galactic center. You know it takes millions of years for a single rev. Yet here you are, a mere spec running down a grassy hillside overlooking the sea. Your energy is here and now. Every cell in your body, every one of those trillions, is tuned to the same energy.

Each breath is an internal moment as you hear the songs of the birds, see the leaves fluttering in the trees, smell the honeysuckle carried on the sea breeze, and feel the effort of the body. Each foot strike is a balanced act in throwing inertia down the hillside with grace. The speed is exciting. The deep breathing is exhilarating. The merging sense of the inner and outer worlds, the "knowing" of all around you, comes from a resonance in the heartbeat.

BOOM, BOOM, BOOM goes the heart.

Sending out a vibration.

BOOM, BOOM, BOOM goes the heart.
Sending out a force from deep within.

BOOM, BOOM, BOOM goes the heart.
Sending out your essence.

BOOM, BOOM, BOOM goes the heart.

*Sending out a force that has always
been with you.*

*A force you are intensifying now,
with your running.*

It is love.

GIVE YOUR FOOD ATTENTION

It would seem that most diets are focused purely on *what* to eat, some perhaps on *when* to eat. But are we missing some basic and important aspects to eating? What about looking beyond the *what* we eat and *when* we eat and into the *how*, *where*, and *why* we eat?

The enormous diet industry and its billions of dollars are almost entirely focused on the *what* and *when* of eating. The best ones keep it super simple, and that's good because it is super simple. Yet, just like running with poor posture will never allow you to find the proper balance and timing, eating the *right* food while not being aware of *how* and *why* you are eating will not allow you to optimize your nutrition.

Diving into the *how* and *why* you eat brings up that same aspect that is being discussed with running throughout this book. Growing the "awareness muscle." Another way for being mindful/ heartful when you eat.

Just like you should apply yourself fully to running, apply yourself fully to eating. You would assume being intrinsically motivated to eat would be simple, and it is, but many in today's society are too distracted to take part. Start with the simple fact that you love eating. Then you can love the food you eat. Now, eat with intention. Give your food the intention of being healthy. Consider the life of the food you are eating. Be grateful for its nourishment. Let the food be thankful to be entering your temple and promise to use it to grow.

Being intrinsically motivated to eat sounds simple enough, but many or most in society are eating for external reasons. Eating for some sort of reward or simple craving of pleasure. Eating emotionally to fill holes and voids left from other aspects of life. Other aspects of life that might be out of control. But eating, you know, is something we can control. When eating is a substitute for any of the emotions based in fear—depression, anxiety, anger—then imagine the intent you are giving the food entering your body. You can send that vibe into the very food you are using to build, repair, and maintain your body.

Other external eating avenues are being distracted. How many people eat with screens staring at them? You can only have so much appreciation for your food when this level of distraction is taking place. Some people sit down and *run a program* (reflexively running a program that is mechanical and mindless) that probably gathered strength in school for a plethora of reasons; eating fast and eating unconsciously being core among them. The *program* is being played by the autonomic nervous system and very little conscious awareness happens. You have seen this in others: they sit down, most likely with poor posture, and eat quickly. Like it is some chore that deserves little or no attention.

Growing the awareness muscle is attention training. Showing up for your meal with your body, mind, heart, and soul puts a powerful dynamic into your eating. What sort of relationship do you have with your food? How do the mind and body in particular relate to each other and the food that you are putting in your temple?

Allow conscious intent to empower your innate gifts. This is so simple that many overlook the profound impact. Let your food assist with your purpose in a way that allows the process to be enjoyed. Eating is a wonderful process. Are you eating in full and absolute awareness? Are you showing up for the meal?

Just like you have a relationship with running via the feedback from your mind, body, heart, and soul complex, the same goes for eating. Here are some potential paths for enhancing and amplifying this relationship. The goal is growth using a beginner's mind. In order to accomplish this, you will need energy, and eating optimally will be integral to your foundation.

It is no coincidence that all the major religions of the world say a prayer before eating. You do not need to be faithful to recognize this benefit. Dr. Masuro Emoto was able to show in reproducible studies that giving intention with your consciousness to water can affect the molecular structure of the water! Amazing. In a classic study reproduced around the world, he took two glasses of water and sealed them. One was given the intention of love while the other was given anger. When the water was frozen and the crystals were examined under a microscope, the differences were startling. The angry water had a distorted and unbalanced crystalline structure, while the water of love had a symmetrically balanced crystalline structure. The water given angry intent looked disagreeable, while the water given love intent was beautiful.

Consider this: You are made up mostly of water. The food you eat is made up of water. You drink water daily. The earth herself is 70 percent water. What kind of message are you sending the water? Science shows that water has memory. Water can retain an imprint of the energies around it.

Is this the reason, is this why all the world's religions know that you should pray before each meal? An innate knowledge passed down through the ages?

All this to say that when you eat, give your food and water the intent. Appreciate your food and the process it took to arrive on your fork. With this intent coming from the heart, you will love the process and your body will show the signs of this process. Eat with heartfulness.

If you eat healthy foods but are not enjoying them, your body will not utilize all the nourishment they contain. Perhaps you are thinking about vitamins, minerals, or calorie count as you eat and are lost in a mental world rather than savoring the taste and enjoying the sensual experience of eating? It cannot be overstated the importance of giving your food the intent and gratitude while being in a state of harmony. Sounds similar to another approach…

Just like you love running…you love your food and you love to eat. Enjoy it.

Part of the message of this book is to take the heartfulness you apply to running and apply it to other parts of your life. Remember, wherever attention goes, energy flows. Give your food attention. Realize this simple task, attention training while you are eating, is a path you will follow the rest of your life. Enjoy the sights, sounds, and smells along the way.

One powerful way to eat is with the breath. It brings awareness to the table. Breathe with the diaphragm and find a calming sensation that comes over the body. Breathe well to deliver oxygenated red blood cells, all 30 trillion of them, to all the other cells of the body. Breathing is an enormous component to keeping the transportation systems in the body open and flowing. You do not want bumper-to-bumper traffic inside the body. Breathing keeps the roadways open for delivery.

With excellent breathing comes excellent posture. You cannot breathe well without also having dignified posture. These two steps are wonderful tricks to help you in overriding old programs (eating fast and/or mechanically). With enough attention training, a day will come where this will be your new default. You will notice more enjoyment in your eating. With this comes more appreciation. Then, better health. And now we have better running, the icing on the cake.

Now that you are breathing well and sitting with centered posture, many of the other best practices for *how* you eat align naturally. If you are at this stage of enjoyment with your meals, you will want to set the table and be free from distractions. You will not only be present and engaged with your food but with the people you are sharing the meal with.

Try something to illustrate the immediate impact of breathing well with good posture. Sit or stand with your best, most dignified posture and belly breathe. Now, try to be depressed. Find it odd or difficult? Now try the opposite. Slump over, slouch, and sit or stand with poor and weak posture. Now try to be happy.

The point is your posture has a huge effect on your energy and attitude.

With a centered presence, it will now be much easier to chew your food. To really chew and chew and chew your food. Do your digestive system a favor and break down the food in your mouth completely. Not only does this help with absorption and getting nutrients to the cells, but it also helps you slow down, be more appreciative, and drop into a deeper level of awareness.

After you give your food and water intent, you begin the same steps you would with running. Take the steps for attention training so you can expand your awareness muscle. Breathe well to have good posture to be centered and focused on your meal. Be present for your meal. If you are sharing it with someone, be with them in silence or in conversation.

This is the most powerful way to eat. Do not eat distracted, do not eat without awareness, do not eat without intention, and do not eat mindlessly or mechanically. In this way, you are not dieting and focusing on what you cannot eat and what you should restrict. Instead, enjoy your food, know your food and, most of all, be present and appreciate your food.

When you do this, you will slow down and eat your food with grace. You will chew your food and savor it. You will listen to your body and know when it is satiated. You will know the cravings your body has for the nutrients it seeks. Imagine the food and water you eat as fortunate to be entering an aware and growing human being that will utilize the energy for love. Reward yourself and others (kids) for eating slowly and listening to the body while you eat.

In doing this, you will achieve all the benefits you seek from dieting and begin to have a relationship with the sustenance you put in your body.

If you cannot know the life of your food, if you cannot appreciate the process it took to arrive at your fork, then why are you eating and supporting a system that has little to no

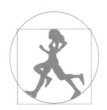

Eat food that is created in a **sustainable** system, a **thriving** system; do this for the future runners of the world.

appreciation for the content of the food? Much of the food produced is for profit and not for the redeeming qualities of nutrition. The entire process must be enjoyed all the way back to the soil and the water that is feeding the food that you eat.

It is one thing to eat food that has little life or nutritional value (this is only harming *you*). It is another to support a system that is not healthy for the environment and the planet at large. In this way, you are harming much more than just yourself in the process of eating industrialized food. If you have a tough time doing it for yourself, then do it for the ones you love and Mother Earth. Eat food that is created in a sustainable system, a thriving system; do this for the future runners of the world. Consider the future seven generations, as in the Native American Indian tradition, and know the best path to take.

Along the path of running, you will grow in appreciation of the relationship you have with the food that energizes and revitalizes your body. To respect and appreciate your food, you will have to respect and appreciate everything that goes into your food: earth, air, and water.

With this as your guide, you will know what to eat, when to eat, and how to eat. Experiment and discover what works best with you. There are as many ways to eat healthy as there are families.

As noted only briefly earlier, consider the life of your food. Yes, every aspect of the life of your food. Living food is the best to eat; we all know you want your food "fresh." This is one aspect, but also consider the treatment and life cycle of your food. Did the plant or animal you are consuming have a good life, a thriving life? This is more than just a passing consideration for the health of your food and therefore your ability to energize and heal with your running. It is also about having a thriving planet to run on.

In this way there are two major aspects to consider when purchasing your food. Your money, for one, is a vote. When you buy something, you are voting for the process that supports it. The obvious aspect of buying healthy food is because it is good for you. But the more important reason to cast your vote carefully is that you are supporting a whole system and process that resonate a thriving life for you and everyone else that shares the planet.

Food for thought: Are you purchasing food that supports a system not just for sustainability but for thriving? You can be pretty certain that when you buy (vote for) processed, industrialized, fast food with lots of packaging, you are supporting a system of destruction for yourself (the food did not have a good life and therefore the life energy is weak), but more importantly the planet.

Use your vote wisely and spend your money on a system that will support growth for you and the planet.

You already know *what* to eat. Michael Pollan sums it up beautifully with seven words: "Eat food, not too much, mostly plants." For some it will be helpful to add, "Eat *real* food." Is your food fresh and prepared simply? Or is it processed, refined, and packaged? Do you understand the entire preparation process? In other words, was the soil treated well that fed the plants that perhaps fed the animals that you are eating? What about the water that fed the soil, plants, and animals? And what about the company you are buying food from? Is that company solely concerned with making money or being a part of a thriving planetary system? Do you know how to pronounce the ingredients? By appreciating and knowing your food, now you can eat with total presence and awareness with gratitude for its nutrients.

If you are not sold on eating food for yourself that you know is good for you, consider the angle mentioned earlier. Your money is a vote. When you purchase something, you are sending a message (I support this, I want more of this), and you keep this process going. When you purchase food from a system that treats the soil, plants, and/or animals poorly, you are supporting the system that is in large part contributing to a more difficult place for children to live and thrive in.

Spend your money wisely; consider what sort of system you are voting for. You would see real and immediate impact for positive change if, in one day, people stopped purchasing food from a system that does not support healthy food.

Do not get stuck on the *what* to eat. You already know what you should eat. Keep it simple and focus on what you can eat instead of what you cannot eat.

This gives you some simple and yet powerful ways for the *what*, *why*, and *how* of eating.

Now, consider *when* to eat in more depth. Have you ever gone for a run where your gut was not ready or still working on a meal that just had not settled yet? It can ruin your run. Having cramps or bloating from the gut can stop you in your tracks or slow you down substantially. In this way, running can be a magnifying glass for the timing and the amount of food you consume.

While racing, the timing and amount of food become critical for your performance. You have to consider the before, during, and after aspects and not forget the importance of how, why, and what you eat while racing—a whole other approach compared to meals at the table.

If you eat the right kind of food and the right amount, it is not difficult to go for a run shortly after a meal. It is not a good time to go for an intense run most likely, but it should not be upsetting to your stomach. Experiment with this to discover the foods that work best for your body.

For performance and intense efforts, it is most likely best to run on an empty stomach, or not have eaten much in the last couple of hours. Food in your gut means energy and blood in your gut that will take away from either your running or the digestive process, both of which will result in less-than-ideal running or digesting.

When eating and running, there is much to consider with regard to the timing and the type and the amount of food. This is unique to each individual. Explore what works in your daily training. The most important aspect is to give your eating the intent it deserves and then to be fully present with the heart while you eat.

Pay attention and show up for your meals. The same way you will pay attention and show up for your runs. By remaining in the present moment, you decrease stress and better recognize your hunger signals. By appreciating your food and sensing the aroma, taste, texture, and colors of the food (while being aware of the whole experience and connecting with those sharing the meal with you), the meal will be upgraded for satisfaction, balance, and health.

Keeping eating simple is just a matter of being ready to free your mind and have an honest relationship between the body and mind. Whatever the cue, being more mindful in one activity can assist in transferring it to any activity. This is simple, yet it is not easy. When this simple aspect of eating naturally and intuitively is applied, the effects are profound.

Consider the following steps each time you eat.

1. Plug in. No distractions. Give your mind and body a break from your day-to-day activities and "set the table" for a dignified meal. Clear away any clutter, noise, and screens. Get away from electronics, and instead connect with someone or enjoy the act of connecting with the food you are about to eat.

2. Breathe. With aware breathing (the next chapters will go into greater detail to expand your awareness of breathing), shift to the present moment. Now you are sending a signal to the entire body and flooding the system with oxygen carrying red blood cells that will be delivering nutrients throughout the entire body. With good breathing comes an aligned posture. Breathing well will reduce any stress and assist you in appreciating your meal.

3. Show intent. By appreciating your food, consider the entire life cycle of the food, and be grateful to have nutrients entering your body. A good way to do this is to say, "Thank you, nature, for the nourishment."

4. Eat slowly. Breathing well will allow slow eating to happen naturally, but make a conscious effort to savor the food. Being the slowest eater at the table is a good rule of thumb. By chewing well and enjoying the flavors, you are starting the digestion process. Pause between bites. Not only will this be much more satisfying, you will notice the moment you are approaching satiation and fullness.

5. Notice your senses. Not just your taste buds. But by all means enjoy the smells and aromas and the sliding scales of bitterness and sweetness. But all your senses should be on high while eating. Listen. Look. Feel. Observe and absorb the meal to its fullest potential by allowing your senses to be activated and used.

6. Understand your relationship with food. By having an open and honest relationship between the body and mind, you can listen and intuitively know your hunger. This will allow you to know

when and how much to eat. Understand that this is a sliding scale from day to day based on many variables. It is a scale that you can listen to and know from day to day and moment to moment better than anyone else.

5

MEASURE YOUR
WELL-BEING (MQ)

By growing your ability to pay attention to something as simple as your movement, you will infuse meaning and therefore expand your well-being. Separate the difference between thinking about your motion and simply being aware of your motion. At first, you will have to think about a new ability, but with practice and focus, your skill expands into awareness. This is a state of Being. Being able to sense beauty is a marker for truth.

When you are aware of meaningful motion, you will not only see but feel this beauty. This is a way of paying attention. Learning the lessons and choosing the right paths will enable the harmony and wisdom you seek. The discernment takes an attitude and imagination born from paying attention with an awareness above mere thinking. An awareness that aligns the body, mind, heart, and soul into a singular focus.

Is there a more powerful human act than one connected to that primal pulse of the heart? An act born from truth and beauty? An act of motion centered with meaning?

THE SHIFT

The constant flow from the snowmelt soothes the ears and, at times, is indistinguishable from the wind flying, swirling, and dancing with the tall pines. An occasional creak from stressed trunks of long-ago dead trees is the only sharp vibration to contrast the soft and silent sounds of the wilderness. Your family is descending the side of a mountain with the youngest setting a wild pace. It came on suddenly, as he shifted from needing a nap to running down the needle-laden single track.

The hike began hours earlier with four adults coercing two young ones into charging up a mountain in the name of fun. A tricky balance between supporting the moment, enjoying the walk, and keeping it alive. Five minutes in and one of the kids is already murmuring about being tired and, "How far are we going?" Although it is not about the destination, it is helpful to have a carrot. "Let's look for a good place to have a picnic." The hike continues with a curi-

osity for rocks, boulders, sticks, mushrooms, and flowers. Each a potential delay in what is usually the adults' steady progress forward. Today, this "want" subsides in order to come alongside the children. To meet them where they are, to encourage the curiosity, to abide by the fact that the journey is the destination.

Everyone gets lost in the play. The play that only those with fresh eyes can see, where nothing is known and everything is a possibility, a discovery. There are boulders and patches of snow to linger in, to lose time in. The laughter comes in bursts as shoes come off and bare feet meet the last of the season's snow.

All six hikers are alive in the moment, lost in the moment, while moving through the wilderness. A hike that never began and never ended, a hike that just is. A dream, a memory, an experience?

The adults played their cards well and supported the kids on a hike that pushed their boundaries without them knowing it. But then it's time to turn around, and it is a long way back. The young ones are rightly tired, and it would seem they will need to be shouldered back down.

Then the shift happens. The gentle grade of the switchbacks makes for fun running, and the kids start flying. The trees flicker in a blur with shouts of joy. Wa-hooo! This image imprints on the mind for eternity. Two children running with such ease, in such beauty that time slows down. It has to—when the mind merges with the heart and allows the soul to take in the total expanse of life. As though the senses are on high alert and processing everything an order of magnitude higher, knowing each of the senses intimately. The conscious slowing down of time is a love for the moment.

The sense of purpose, the joy in seeing others thrive, the subtle energy coming alive in the wilderness melts their whole Being. A shared instant in time that lingers all the way down the mountain. This is when motion takes them beyond the motion. This motion can be a gateway. It is a gateway that the children know well, if only the adults are receptive enough to let the children show the way.

DEFINING MQUOTIENT (MQ)

"Walking is man's best medicine."

—*Hippocrates*

MQuotient3 (MQ3) = Motion Quotient x Mindful Quotient x Meaning Quotient

MQ= Well-Being

MQuotient (MQ) stands for Motion Quotient, Mindful Quotient, and Meaning Quotient. Similar to IQ (intelligence quotient) and EQ (emotional quotient), MQ references three areas of measurement (motion, mindfulness, and meaning) multiplied to reveal your overall well-being. MQ is about coming alongside you and starting a journey by understanding and activating all of the abilities you will need to empower your best performance in every action.

In only a few short minutes, your MQ score can be determined, and while the score itself will be telling, it is the discernment of the test to help you establish an awareness of how best to ensure and improve your own well-being.

**To learn more and find out your own MQ score, please
visit my website www.mqscore.com.**

Like learning to read and write, your ability to move with
meaning is teachable. Would we leave a stack of books, papers,
and pens, and just assume that a child is going to learn to read
and write on his own? Certainly not. We have experts to work
with and progress children through years of practice. But what
about mobility? What about teaching the foundations for human
movement? Sure, a few learn these skills through sports, but
we have many who are not exposed, and even the ones who
are exposed mistake human movement for some sort of hyper-
competition. And what about walking? When was the last time
you considered *how* you walk? Two years old?

Motion is a big deal; you understand this on one level but
ignore it on another. Celebrating the majesty of the sports heroes,
putting them in an iconic class, above and beyond the rest of
humanity. Thinking and treating them like super beings. But
what about everybody else, the other 99.99 percent of humanity?
Is there a way to close this gap, to have the rest of humanity
appreciate and practice and grow their ability to understand their
unique Motion Quotient?

Your ability to move well goes far beyond just competing in
sports. It is a foundation for everything you will do in life. True
Wealth can only be achieved with optimizing your aptitude for
breathing well through moving well. Mental health and physical
health are married. It is only when both of these characteristics
are motivated that one can reach their true potential and their
True Wealth is realized.

Motion Quotient. Have you considered your ability to move? You know it is teachable, something that requires practice to master. It is nothing more than an awareness. Just like IQ or EQ, it is simply another tool to measure someone's awareness. The more aware you are of intelligence, emotions, or movements, the better you will perform. How might we measure humanity in its understanding and ability to move? How might we teach it? There are ways to measure a very limited angle of intelligence with IQ, but many view a high EQ as a more valuable skill. Fact is, there are many components to intelligence. Consider: visual, musical, verbal, logical, body, interpersonal, intrapersonal, naturalistic, existential, teaching, and humor. What is the value of such measurements but having the ability to assess and assist someone with his unique, next best step? The real value is the ability to use the tool to begin a dialogue to connect with mentors who can work on their teaching angle of intelligence and shift people in a positive direction.

The point is, MQ is not fixed. It is not something you are born with; it is not limited to your genes. No, MQ mastery takes experience and teaching. The accurate use of an MQ is merely to determine where on the sliding evolution of well-being a person is and then apply, through supportive teaching, the right awareness cards for this unique individual to pay attention to. In this way, they can improve in the most enjoyable way possible.

MQ is a simple tool to measure the intelligence of the body and the kinesthetic aptitudes. How well do you move; how aware are you of your motions? This is not something that we should limit to the athletes, dancers, and soldiers of the world. Just like there is a massive effort to teach the skills of reading and writing, the skills of movement should be held with the same esteem. The world is facing an epidemic, a health crisis that has a lot of smart people trying to figure out solutions. There is a common thread that can cut across all of the issues, from diabetes and heart disease, to cancer, obesity, and mental health. Here is a simple solution: teach MQ. Make the process innovative and exciting and something that is practiced with focus, day in and day out—because it is fun.

Having mentors who can shift people's MQ is simple, and here is how to do it. Wait for it, drum roll please…keep the drum roll, wait for it…by walking. "What!?" "Walking!?" you say. "I figured that out when I was two, and I have that down, just like everyone else."

Wrong.

You are taking your ability to walk for granted. Most of the world pays little attention to walking well, does not know what a good walk is, and does not know that on the sliding scale of measuring walking, they are on the poor end of it. Matter of fact, apart from a few isolated communities where walking knowledge is passed down and valued, the rest of the world gets a failing mark for its ability to walk well. Some may be fair walkers, but very few are doing well and almost no one is doing great.

What if you gained some insight, if someone gave you an edge, an edge for knowing and understanding how to walk supreme? What if, from that moment of understanding, you took every step for the rest of your life…and each was a little bit better? How might this affect your life? Consider all the paths.

You will have the energy and therefore the curiosity to discover and take more paths. You will be able to travel the paths farther than before. And, with each step you take, you will notice more, feel more, and experience more because you are simply more aware. Consider this important question again: How might your life be affected if every step you take from now on is better? What might this do for your well-being?

What if the *art* in the heart of running is all about walking? What if walking lays the foundation for something more to happen? What if walking is the most important door to open to discover mastery of all human motions?

By playing the cards you acquire with an MQ, which at its foundation is walking, you will know how **mindfulness** is the key component to making the choice to pay attention. By expanding this ability to pay attention to your **motion,** you gain a sense of purpose; you move with **meaning**.

Do you know of anyone who was formally taught how to walk? Is there a program that passes along the knowledge of best practices from years and generations of walking? There are speed walkers, but that is a different discussion. Consider this: You can see the stark difference of a formal versus self-taught swimmer. In the early days of swimming, athletes basically were self-taught. The world record from Johnny Weissmuller (Tarzan) in 1922 is 58.6 seconds in the 100-meter freestyle. Today, the U.S. national record in the same event for 11- and 12-year-old boys is 55.03. For girls it is 56.87. This is just an example of having knowledge of best practices and formal teaching of a craft. Johnny didn't have many, if any, experts to tap into back in 1922. If someone back in 1922 simply had the knowledge that thousands of swim coaches have today, a 12-year-old girl could have out-swum the entire world.

Today, the best walkers are like Tarzan—they are self-taught. And while they might be doing it well as compared to the rest of the public, that does not mean they are optimized. Swimming progressed because coaches learned from the best and taught all the rest what they were doing. Then one of those students took it to another level. Then the next coach learned from the best and taught all the rest, and so goes The Way. This is not happening in walking at all…and everyone walks!

You can become a decent swimmer by playing and being self-taught, but a very young boy or girl with some formal swimming education and practice will swim circles around you. But, of course, this is not entirely the point for walking. It is not so much about walking fast; it is about walking well and infusing your motion with all the health you are capable of. There is a worrying trend that is happening as societies across the globe morph from what is now becoming far-removed walking societies to sitting ones. With no formal education and very little pass down of the knowledge of best practices for walking, the best of the self-taught walkers today seem to be worse than the ones a few decades ago. How far has humanity slid in walking? Is there the chance humanity will lose its knowledge of supreme walking if the current trends continue? Yes!

Here is a little-known secret. Humans are very good at walking. NO, not the less-than-half activated walk you see happening all over the globe, but a human walking with awareness—a human

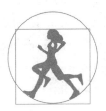

Today, the best walkers
are like Tarzan—**they are
self-taught.**

walking supreme. For most it only takes minutes to activate, upgrade, and turn on the whole body motion of a human walking well. For whatever the reason, one of your main walking switches is in the "off" position. It does not take much to flip the switch "on." With the right cues, people can transform their walking to include the natural swagger they were born with. It takes minutes to understand and emulate. Then, depending on your age, it takes days, weeks, and months to unlearn old habits. Once you are mindful to notice, you give yourself the opportunity to grow your awareness for an upgraded walk.

The foundation for movement comes from walking. Yet after we learned to walk at a very young age, through much trial and error, we rarely—if ever—give the form aspect of walking another consideration. This is more than a slight oversight; it is a big deal. Few people are actually walking with desirable form. There is more to walking than simply having good posture and walking tall.

Regardless of how well you are doing it, walking should be a healthy endeavor. But you want to go beyond sustaining and into thriving. How well do you walk? **Walking at the top level is an art of precision, balance, timing, and grace.** Do you feel the joy, grace, and efficiency of an exceptional walk? No matter your level, there are awareness cards you can play to increase your ability, enjoyment, and performance.

You're skeptical and you should be. You don't know what you don't know. **What does a good or great walk look like? Who is passing along and teaching walking?** These are monumental questions that, for some reason, few have paid attention to lately.

Fortunately, there are skilled people among you who have this knowledge and who are willing and ready to give humanity a slap of reality. Smack! "Wake up and walk with purpose and awareness!" It is simple, not easy, but with a good teacher, people are able to transform from a good to great walker in a matter of minutes. As mentioned, it is almost as if the light switch has been turned off, and all you need to do is flip the awareness switch. Many will wonder, "This is so obvious! Why haven't I activated this?" Almost as if you have been blocking and holding back your abilities. Why? Most cultures of the world have gravitated from a walking culture to a sitting culture. The high-level walkers are not being activated, not being taught, not being recognized. Walking is no longer valued.

To walk well, you need to have well-developed feet and hips to be able to have dynamic balance. Using the foot as it has been designed for each individual is key. Contacting the ground correctly sets in motion a powerful human kinetic guide wire. This allows you to tap into free energy. Being able to contact the ground correctly takes proper hip recruitment. The ground force reaction can be a good or bad stress depending on how your body utilizes motion. If you are an elite athlete, knowing the mechanics for sound walking will transfer directly into your sport. On the other end of the spectrum, if you are using walking for rehabilitation, fitness, or mood enhancement, having the tools to know the correct motions will increase your abilities and your enjoyment tenfold.

You have all heard, "You have to walk before you run." But we have all sidestepped the message, literally and figuratively.

Once you know what to look for in a good walker, you begin looking for someone who is doing it. You just will not see it. Occasionally, you might get a glimpse, but rarely do you see someone walking with awareness.

That zombie apocalypse…it's been here for a long time. Most of humanity is walking around with little attention or awareness of their God-given swagger. It is not a showy swagger, just a human, walking with resolution. Unique to each and every one, but a certain swagger for sure.

There is another aspect of MQ: MQ squared. When you add mindfulness to motion, you amplify the effect greatly. MQ is all about paying attention with the body and mind to let the spirit play. When you mirror a centered and focused mind with an aware and present body, you align yourself with optimal abilities.

Move; move well; it is simple; you just need to pay attention. Or it helps if you read the User Manual? What User Manual? There isn't one. Humans don't come with one, but we can pass down and teach the knowledge.

Well, humans have forgotten to read the first chapter in the User Manual on walking.

That is the nicest way to put it.

You skipped the chapter on walking and went straight to the exciting stuff like jumping and running. But you don't know what you don't know. Who could have imagined that walking could be so powerful and so fun!?

So, the important questions eluded to earlier: What do you think is a good walk? How do you know? What do you look for? Why do you care? How do you define a good walk?

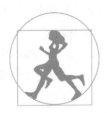

Most of humanity is walking around with little attention or awareness of their **God-given swagger**. It is not a showy swagger, just a human, walking with resolution. Unique to each and every one, but a certain swagger for sure.

And for many the answer is, "I don't know." And that is the most important answer.

Some other questions to consider: Who is teaching our kids how to walk? Who are we emulating? Do we have mentors and role models for sound walking?

Again, a simple answer. Except for a few small circles within cultures, no one is teaching walking. Most of you have not seen a human walking well and therefore have no mentor. Yes, it is crazy. There are billions of humans walking on the planet, and you most likely have not seen a person fully activated in supreme human walking. Many apply the fitness aspect of walking. This is great and very powerful. However, imagine if every step, every breath, and every heartbeat was that much stronger because you are aware of supreme human walking. It is simple, yet not easy.

Here is where you can have a heyday with the health benefits of walking. It is endless and you know it. Every angle of health can be supported through walking.

Now imagine all the people out there looking to improve their health. They go for a walk and it is not fun...for many, it even hurts. They assume a myriad of reasons for why they don't walk well or why they just don't like walking, but none of them assume they are doing it wrong. How does this help those who are trying to mobilize a team, a corporation, or a city into wellness action? It doesn't help much, especially if the main objective is fitness and exercise. These people are just going to throw in the white flag in frustration and tell you they don't care.

On the other end of the spectrum, you have athletes who are not tapping into one of the most powerful tools in their training.

They are missing gaining an edge or performing at their highest level.

Walking pulls, twists, stretches, and rotates the whole body into motion. By whole body, I really am referring to the WHOLE body (mind, body, heart, and soul). Consider the angles of awareness that can be magnified and amplified by walking. From mental clarity to blood flow, to social interaction and sense of purpose. All the angles of the wheel of health can be lit up through supreme human walking. It is almost more of a letting go, a simple letting go, to remember how you are truly meant to walk.

Many of the greatest insights and inventions have come during a downtime, when the inventor, literally and figuratively, stepped away from his work. In this stillness, in this centered walking, in this motion, moving beyond the motion—an epiphany. The lights go on, and an answer appears out of thin air.

At the highest order of walking well is an awareness that brings joy, compassion, and appreciation for the merging of the whole body while you walk. As you upgrade your walking, blood flow happens freely and more completely, delivering feel-good hormones and nutrients to every cell in your body. As you promote your walking, the ability to focus your mind's energy on being creative and innovative is amplified. This alignment of the body and mind opens up your potential.

"All truly great thoughts are conceived while walking."

—Friedrich Nietzsche

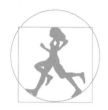

Walking is **sexy**. Walking is the embodiment of mindfulness, and by activating all of your motions, you accelerate your understanding.

Walking is sexy. Walking is the embodiment of mindfulness, and by activating all of your motions, you accelerate your understanding. "What did you just say!?"

Walking is sexy.

"No, the bit after that?"

By paying attention, energy flows to that focus. By growing your attention, you grow your energy.

Another way, as mentioned earlier and said many times by many people, "Wherever attention goes, energy flows." Well, then…grow your attention and increase your energy.

After all, energy management is a lot about time management—which is all about paying attention. When you perform a craft you know well, a craft you know intimately, then you can perform it well. One way to look at the slowing down of time is an increased awareness. Is it not the same thing? How else do you describe the mastery of any craft by any master but the ability to "slow down time" and pay attention to every detail in an effortless way?

This is supreme walking. It is also a path for running. Any and all crafts. Begin the discovery of motion with walking by instilling best practices and then applying this understanding and knowledge to an MQ for running, biking, and swimming. These basic movements, these human-powered ways to move from point A to point B are a great way to play. By laying a foundation for walking, all other activities will be upgraded. You will move better in everything from golf to tennis to basketball to soccer.

Correct walking is essential for continued health and

wellness. Walking is your foundation for thriving and increasing your health and well-being.

MQ is about paying attention to grow your abilities. Learn how to pay attention. Then add another layer and learn how to learn how to pay attention. Learning to learn. It is a path you can never summit. There is always another level. This is "flexing your awareness muscle." This is an attempt to meet people where they are, that this hard "flexing" is the way to pay attention. This is part of the process and the evolution toward moving from a hard concentration to a light but still laser-sharp focus. Consider it, in reality, more of a simple and light stretch than a flex. Now take this mental imagery of stretching instead of flexing and apply it to the body. This is the "magic" of utilizing connective tissue when you walk. It is not about flexing but stretching.

But here lies a major problem. The social construct of walking. The social norms. What a culture accepts as "normal" walking. Don't do this; don't do that. You don't want to stand out too much or be boastful or showy. So many clichés in how to walk, many not true. The text was not entirely truthful about having walkers to emulate in society. There are some out there who have not unlearned yet, some children. But then they enter a system that values sitting quietly over walking purposefully.

It is about a human walking in awareness and performing an activity by activating all of your abilities. Person after person walking around today is not activating many aspects of their walking. When you look at the human figure, you notice all the lines of pull on 45-degree angles. All these "x's" allow for contralateral behavior. Consider the connection of the left arm swinging with the right leg as an example of these lines of pull that cross the center of gravity. Rotation is key. The human form moves best when you activate your lines of pull that create rotational forces. This is torque, balance, efficiency, power, and grace.

Motion at the highest levels is about tapping into the connective tissue, the fascia and myofascia. It is not about muscling it unless you are sprinting, which should last less than a minute. For activities lasting longer than a minute, the key to effective mastery is utilizing and recruiting the connective tissue. Muscle is costly metabolically; it needs blood and oxygen—and lots of it—when moving in a muscling sort of way. Connective tissue does not require lots of blood. Aha! The light just went on.

Flex muscles and they need energy. When blood is circulated, the muscles take the nutrients they are delivering. However, the connective tissue does not. It does not need the nutrients on a second-by-second basis in order to perform. If you can stretch the muscles instead of flexing them, now they are not nearly as costly in terms of their need for energy. A muscle in stretch is more like a pulsing heart. A muscle in stretch does not need blood as much as it can help pump blood around the body. Imagine a body utilizing 100 hearts instead of one!

You see, by using the "x's" and these connective tissues, you are shrink-wrapping the muscles and using subtle and light stretching to move the body effectively. Now, instead of the muscles desperately asking for shipments of blood, they are acting like another heart and are helping the heart pulse blood throughout the body.

This stretch is pretty easy for people to implement while walking. By applying this mobility to the body, by taking weeks and months to remodel the body with this new stimulus, the effects are compounded. As your awareness grows and your body adapts, your body and mind remodel. You upgrade the human form. You will notice it in everything you do. Now you have the key to stretching in something simple but more difficult than walking; take running for example.

The key to all of this is to be excited about practicing. To know how and what to pay attention to, and then to do it often. If you are having fun, it will be the most natural thing in the world.

You cannot just read about walking; it must be experienced the same as parachuting and bungee jumping. Through conditioning and flexing your awareness muscle, you can learn to upgrade your subconscious walking all the time, even when you are not aware of it, and your autonomic nervous system takes over. This takes mindfulness. In fact, it is about 66 days of thought focus before you can simply be aware and perform effortlessly.

The power of walking is severely underestimated by many. Not just the physical stamina obtained from it but also the alignment with purpose, meaning, and clarity from breathing a little deeper and increasing blood flow while calming the mind. As Mr. Nietzsche and others have stated, walking is a wonderful **way to increase insight, innovation, and creativity**.

Walking *IS* sexy. Consider the stimulating, exciting, sensual, deep breathing that can be maintained for long periods of time. Walking is an instinctual drive and, by optimizing it, you activate the WHOLE body by triggering movement. Purposeful movement.

You know walking is awesome, but imagine for a moment if you could take every single step just a little bit better. What might you do, what might be enhanced if every step you take from this moment onward could be improved?

"But how do I do it? What do I need to unlearn? What do I pay attention to?"

Here are some aspects to consider (and these are benefits for a large percentage of the people walking just okay or poorly).

WALKING BENEFITS:

- Slows down the aging process
- Means you are not sitting, which is worse for you than smoking
- Reduces the risk of coronary heart disease
- Improves blood pressure and sugar levels
- Improves blood lipid profile
- Maintains body weight and lowers the risk of obesity
- Enhances mental well-being
- Reduces your risk of osteoporosis
- Reduces your risk of breast and colon cancer
- Reduces your risk of non-insulin dependent (type 2) diabetes
- Increases your ability to rehab and recover
- Increases your exposure to nature and sunlight
- Improves clarity, creativity, and innovation

- Improves concentration and focus
- Increases energy levels
- Reduces stress
- Regulates fasting glucose levels among people with diabetes
- Reduces the effects of rheumatoid arthritis, hypertension, PMS, chronic muscle and joint pain, asthma and respiratory conditions
- Increases immune system activity and response
- Strengthens feet and hips

HERE'S HOW:

If you had a User Manual for supreme human walking, the chapters might cover these areas (note: this is just one way of many to discover the principles of sound walking):

1. Locomotor: from the top of the hips (iliac crest) down
2. Passenger: from the top of the hips up
3. Posterior Guide Wires: the connective tissue from head to toe along the backside
4. Anterior Guide Wires: the connective tissue from the jaw to the toes along the front side
5. Spiral Motors: activating the rotational components of the whole body

Each of these five areas of the body has many aspects to consider within them but also include how they interact with each other. The human body is one long connection from head to toe. If you move something on the left, chances are it affects something on the right. If you move something at the top, chances are you affect something at the bottom. Then reflect on how the body moves in 3D. Many study, teach, and think of the body as moving in 2D, but being aware of the 3D component and all of its gyrations is the way to truly understanding human motion.

Beginning with the locomotor and the hips, very few people are initiating the walk with the control center, the fulcrum, the holy grail of motion that lies in the hips. The pelvis should be rotating; it is known in some circles as lead change. Lead change the hips by allowing the right hip to come forward with the right heel striking the ground. On the other side of the equation, the left hip is rotated back to delay the toe off. You can only focus on the front or back aspect of this motion to begin with, but essentially it is the same motion. This lead change of the hips activates something that has been dormant in many: the spinal motor. It is only half of the spinal motor, but it is a powerful form of efficiency, balance, and grace to upgrade your walking abilities.

Add to this a pelvis rotation within a rotation. The ilium can rotate as well. While the pelvis is rotating on the z-axis (the left to right heading), the ilium can rotate the pitch on the x-axis (up or down). This is a powerful way to increase the length of the pole vault that is a straight leg at heel strike. Let the right hip rotate forward (z-axis) at heel strike while allowing the ilium to rotate backwards (on the x-axis/pitch). These create a longer leg to increase the torque of the pole vault.

Very few are walking with much—if any—rotation in the hips, instead, choosing to hold a position incorrectly.

Another important aspect of the locomotor was already mentioned in explaining the pelvis rotations. Yes, in walking, you want to heel strike, and you want to heel strike with a straight leg. Coupled with a rotating pelvis, this lengthens the gait without flexing or adding resistance. Matter of fact, it can smooth out the resistance by transforming it into potential and kinetic energy!

Meeting the ground force with a straight leg allows the ground force reaction to travel up the leg to the glutes. These big and powerful muscles are there for this purpose. To absorb and utilize the ground force. But it only happens if the leg is straight at impact.

Now, look at how the foot and ankle should interact with the ground force. After meeting the ground with the calcaneus (heel bone), roll it toward the little toe. Many will go from the heel straight to the big toe stressing out anything from the foot, to the ankle, to the knee. The correct motion is to go from the heel and rock to the little toe. Then use the transverse arch and rock toward the big toe.

An easy and insightful illustration of this is to drum roll with your hand and fingers. Meet a surface with the wrist (heel) and then drum roll beginning with the little finger (little toe) and work over to the thumb (big toe) to have the whole hand (foot) on the ground. These three points form the triangulation that gives the foot the most support and allows for you to pronate into the main arch of your foot. This is important. Once these three triangulating points are flat on the ground, your ankle has rolled forward to bring the full weight of your body onto your foot. This is a crucial moment. A chance to activate your spring ligament. It is actually called the spring ligament, and you probably haven't used it much in your motion.

If you look at a lateral view of the foot and narrow in on the arch, there is a pyramid with the spring ligament being the keystone at the top of the pyramid. At the base is the plantar fascia, then, in the middle, is the long and short plantar ligaments, and at the top is the spring. The only way to activate the spring is to dig into your arch with a natural pronation and...spring. This happens with the full weight of your body centered over the spring, an instant after the foot is flat on the surface.

These are a few elements to consider when looking into the human locomotor. There are more, of course, but it is best to meet with a walking coach or an MQ specialist to discover and play with other components of the locomotor.

The passenger is above the hips, and most of the world is walking with a static passenger. The passenger is dead weight. Here is how to activate and assist the whole body in walking with a triggered passenger.

Rotate.

Your spine can rotate at three areas: your neck (C1 to C7), your thoracic cage, rib cage (T1 to T12) and your lumbar (L1 to L5). Each area can rotate independent of the other and even in opposite directions. This is a key component to the spinal motor.

Take a moment and rotate each area of the spine by itself. You should have no problem rotating the neck without moving anything else. Many will have a tougher time rotating the rib cage without affecting the neck or hips, but you will find it possible with practice. The lumbar is more of a stabilization that allows the hips to rotate without affecting the rib cage.

To flip the switch and activate the passenger, simply allow and recruit the rib cage to rotate. Do not hold a still position. The arm swing will show you the timing. When you begin rotating from T12 up, the arm swing will be happening more from the rotation of rib cage than from engaging the shoulders.

A key aspect to this rotation is that you can focus on rotating forward or backward. It is essentially the same motion, but by focusing your attention on pushing the scapula area backward, people will hold a better head position.

This rib cage activation is a powerful stretch. You will feel the guide wires being pulled in 45-degree "x's." Consider just a few: the right shoulder to the left hip (best felt when the right shoulder is rotating backwards). The right latissimus dorsi (lat) to the left glutes (best felt when the right lat is rotating forward). The right oblique muscles to the left psoas major (best felt when the left leg is delaying at toe off).

The posterior guide wires are a way to reflect on the connective tissue that begins just above your eyebrows and wraps around the skull and then has two main sections that run along each side of the spine and each leg until it wraps underneath the heel of the foot.

If you lean forward, you are making all these posterior guide wires tight. Imagine what happens when you tune the strings of a guitar too tightly. First, you can't play beautiful music. Second, you might fray or even snap a wire. In the human body, this makes you tight and ill at ease to move gracefully.

The posterior and anterior guide wires work together and in balance if the body has sound posture and a close-fitting lateral line equating to a small center of gravity. Stand tall and bend at the waist. Where is your center of gravity? It becomes a wide area in front of your hips. Stand tall with good posture and you can feel and know the precise point where the center of gravity is importantly under your pelvis.

The point is that by finding the right tension for the anterior and posterior guide wires, you have a center of gravity located precisely under your hips with your head directly over it. Many people have a tight posterior guide wire simply because the head is leaning forward and in front of the center of gravity. The fix is not to jolt the neck backwards, although the neck position may need to be played with. The fix is to allow some slack in the posterior guide wires by allowing the natural "c" in the lumbar/lower back and coupling that with a proud chest where the shoulders are square. This often will allow the ears to be over the shoulder, which are over the hips, knees, and ankles when standing with correct posture. While walking, simply look for the ears to be over the shoulders.

What happens to the anterior guide wires when the posterior is tight? The anterior becomes slack, and hence, the ability of the front of the body to manipulate and control motion is severely compromised. Over time, slack anterior guide wires can no longer hold the front of the body's shape and this slack can be evident in the belly.

When the locomotor, passenger, anterior, and posterior guide wires are all triggered, the spinal motor can come online with all the gears and power it has to offer. Much of it is almost free energy. The gyration forces created by the pelvis and thoracic cage rotating counter to each other offer up a plethora of feel-good motions that turn into powerful emotions. These counter forces working together initiate a balance and a grace as well as an ease of effort for human-powered movement. This is but a glimpse of the wonders of walking and some areas for you to focus on.

A trained MQ expert can transform a person's walk in about 30 minutes. That is mostly a testament to how well humans are walking and "remembering" their supreme motions. There are a million ways to walk, and you will have your own unique style and way of doing it. The key is to know all the systems available to you and to flip them on; initiate a whole body walking. Initiate a human walking with awareness. You will see and feel the inner smile. The potential for this inner smile is the compassion that you will grow for yourself and others.

Consider a future planet, one not too far off, one that your children inherit. If there were a million planets in the Milky Way galaxy and one way to assess the advancement of a civilization was the walkability of the planet, how would earth fair today? Is the planet aligned with paths for humans to walk, experience, play, socialize, discover, explore, mingle, and blend with nature? What about through the heart of a city? Do you live in a walkable city? What might one, the best one, look like? And what comes first, a walkable city or the walker?

How might that city with supreme walkability compare in

terms of human productivity? What kind of shift might happen? To feel the earth under your feet and to transcend the motion, to go beyond the motion through something as simple as walking.

If you can fall in love with walking, if you can support others in falling in love with their walking, what kind of world might that create? What would a world full of people who love to walk and who enable others to do the same look and feel like? Would it amplify the art in the heart of being a human? Does it open the possibility of growing the human qualities we hold dearest? Does it amplify your creativity, innovation, compassion, and love for yourself and others? Imagine a world that loves to walk, then take your next step by living the change you want to see, as Gandhi eloquently taught us.

Walking is with You. Where are You?

Many of the best answers in life propagate from coming to a point where the correct answer lies in discovering the right question.

6a
BREATHING AS A
BRIDGE TO THE SOUL

The NightRunner is a superhero complete with a hidden identity (your normal day-to-day life) who can transform, with a single running breath, into The NightRunner. The NightRunner knows well the cards to play to experience the Runner's High. She can tap into a raw animal instinct that has her alert, alive, and performing at her highest abilities. She loves to run. She loves to run in natural settings and knows well how to appreciate the moment.

In this moment is a stillness and a depth that is rich with feeling.

PRESENT, ALERT, ALIVE

The moon is rising, casting shadows and beckoning for you to drop into the body and breathe deeply. While the rest of the world sits, you activate. A presence comes over you or into you, like you have just occupied your body for the first time all day. You watch your breath as you acquire the necessary gear for the night run. Your senses become alert, hawkishly alert, as you become aware of the dullness of your day up to this point. The uniqueness of running in the dark brings forth a stimulus, a challenge, which your body, mind, and soul welcome. You are not "doing" running or "thinking" running; your whole Being is involved in a dance as one so that you might BE the runner.

Your first running breath completes the transition.

It is not the breath itself, but the cue. The awareness of the breath as it moves from body to mind to soul. The rhythm is known. The balance is exquisite as you find neutral. The sacred neutral in the body brings out a relaxed movement in tune with timing and balance. In the mind, this neutrality brings a peace. A peace born of purpose. Like a thirsty desert plant, the mind drinks in the calm and thanks you for the reprieve from the onslaught of distractions it has endured all day. You run on. You run with power and grace. You watch the body and marvel. You are not concerned with any of the doings of running...not pace, not fitness, not distance, not time. You are simply aware and running.

Running is the trigger for being The NightRunner.

Wake up! You are running.

KNOWING THE BREATH

Throughout the day you resided at the surface of the mind. The surface is like being on a small raft on the Pacific Ocean. Weather comes and goes; storms throw you this way and that as you float on the whims of your external world. Sometimes the sea is still, and yet it is not you controlling the stillness. The storms and waves can be viewed as the emotions and thoughts of the mind. The mind is vast like the Pacific. To find peace and clarity, no matter the weather on the surface, all you need to do is drop down. Just under the surface lies the stillness.

In this stillness you can be aware and be the observer. You can see the surface, but now, with greater depth and transparency, you are not emotionally charged with the surface activities.

"Breath is the bridge, which connects life to consciousness, which unites your body to your thoughts. Whenever your mind becomes scattered, use your breath as the means to take hold of your mind again."

—Thích Nhât Hanh

Another way to talk about the heart of running is to discuss "breath." Knowing your breath is knowing yourself. To be a runner takes exquisite, fluid, life-enhancing breathing. First, you will feel the breath; eventually, you will think the breath with deeper concentration, and then a true understanding will happen as you know the breath. This "knowing" the breath is not about the breath. It is about the awareness of the breath. This opens up your potential, and the possibilities are limitless.

As teacher Nhat Hanh suggests, the breath is the connection between the body and the soul with the mind being the bridge. The mind's true talent comes in its ability to interact with our physical body as well as our spiritual body. In order to do this, the mind cannot be distracted. The mind needs to be alert, open, and ready to receive the soul. This is how the mind can serve the soul. Breathing is a gateway into this understanding. Running is a way to accelerate the process. Running forces a deeper relationship with the breath; running makes you aware of the breath, aware of the instant, each exhale and inhale so vital to sustain the running.

To achieve running flow means the body, mind, and soul are dancing in unison. You are here to do this in your own unique way; running is one of the many paths to aid you in achieving this state.

USING YOUR EMOTIONAL INTELLIGENCE

Emotional intelligence is defined as *the ability to recognize one's own and other people's emotions, to discriminate between different feelings and label them appropriately, and to use emotional information to guide thinking and behavior.* At the heart of being emotionally intelligent is knowing yourself. As mentioned earlier, many in society have their mind servicing their body. Emotional wreck is an understatement. The flood of emotions from the body rule the mind as it reacts and stumbles and distracts. The mind is full of potential, but to serve the body lowers its capacity.

Many have the hierarchy correct with the body serving the mind but leave it to this. The mind is amazing and wonderful, but even the most powerful thinking mind enters a realm far greater than its ability to comprehend the true wonder of the soul. Insight, creativity, new ideas, and concepts are born from the soul whereby the mind is calm to a point of receiving the signal.

The body acts and emits emotions in service to the mind. The mind thinks and focuses emotions in service to the soul. The soul knows and empowers the emotional energy.

To know these connections, to serve these relationships, you need to understand your breathing.

To be a master runner first takes a master breather.

The breath is always with You. Where are You?

Although you are probably unaware of your breathing most of the day—if not all of the day—it is your connection to the life source. The aim of this teaching is to be consciously aware of every breath you take while running, yet the applications are limitless and boundless. Just like the inhale and the exhale.

You will need to become consciously aware of your breath to achieve mastery of any action. At first just a few seconds periodically throughout the day. Eventually you notice an amplification for the activity. You notice an increased ability to be aware and to focus on whatever activity you are doing. With practice you begin to progress to a few minutes periodically throughout the day. The focus is more precise, more efficient. You become able to concentrate more intensely for longer periods of time with less and less effort. During these times of conscious breathing, your alertness goes up, your abilities are refined, you are spontaneous and creative, and your energy is always sufficient.

Eventually, this awareness becomes your natural state. It takes weeks, months, and years stretched out over time to practice and hone your skills. The essence of conscious breathing could be summed up as follows: to relax the body, which assists in relaxing the mind and vice versa. With this calm, still, and peaceful mind and body, with a mind and body in harmony, in sync, and in focus, the soul can be received and accepted and, eventually, heard.

The aim of being mindful—of breathing well—is to prime the mind for a greater presence, that much greater awareness we call the soul. To be able to host our soul is to be in union, to be connected, to be in flow, to obtain a Runner's High.

It can be done by anyone, yet few achieve it. Running is but one path and one you are welcome to join. You have had these moments; something took your breath away, a pure impulse, a timeless moment of recognition, the desire to act beyond the sphere of your own personal interests and motives, in the recognition of another, in the motive to give, in the inexplicable experience of affinity. These moments that may have taken you by surprise are actually your natural state. The mind becomes shell-shocked and stops dominating your awareness. The mind can be tricked into doing what it loves to do: amplify itself to receive and experience a Pure Experience, or what runners like to call a Runner's High.

You can run for years; you can be a track star, an Olympian, even a world champion and not truly know your breathing, but what an opportunity missed, a level of satisfaction lost, and an even greater ability to perform squandered. Perhaps some of the great runners fall into the rhythm by chance; perhaps that is the secret to their greatness. Some are aware of this and some are not. This teaching wants to open that door for you, a door that will open many other doors.

Knowing your breath allows you to be mindful under any situation. Doing the dishes, meditating, changing diapers, running, working, eating, swimming, sitting, listening, anything you do while breathing. So, yes, everything. To maintain awareness, one must watch the breath with a practiced concentration.

You take 15,000 breaths a day if you conservatively assume 10 breaths a minute. Imagine what might happen if you made each breath just a tiny bit better? Fifteen thousand multiplied by a tiny bit is a whole lot. That's just one day. You probably take over 100,000 breaths a week. What if you didn't just make each breath a little bit better but a whole lot better? It is entirely possible and it is simple. The effect can be profound. When you embark on a journey to know and understand your breathing, you can be amazed at how powerful one breath can be. One breath in awareness is worth a million mindless ones. Laying the foundation to upgrade each breath should be something everyone pays attention to. It should be taught with all seriousness and focus (play) to our children. There should be Ph.D.s for breathing.

Ask yourself these important questions: How well do you breathe? Do you know your breath? How often are you aware of your breathing? Take a moment and be aware of your next three breaths.

Did you rush them? Did you enjoy them? Did you feel a reaction?

Consider for a moment how your body is able to be aware of the breathing. Consider how the mind perceives the breathing. Observe the breath and observe the mind and body at sync and in harmony. While doing this in stillness, ask yourself, who is watching the mind and the body? Who!? Who is truly overseeing this orchestra? Many of you stop with the mind, but you must go farther. It takes a stillness of the mind to receive the soul.

Knowing your breath is this stillness. It sounds so simple because it is. Yet if you try to go for a 40-minute run, how many of those breaths will you be aware of? Most people will only last a few breaths. Some may be able to focus for a minute or even a few minutes. If you can focus and know every breath you take for a 40-minute run, then you are well advanced in your understanding. Truth must always bring simplicity. With this simple assessment, you can understand where you are and how much work needs to be done.

Simplicity will bring resolution and profound understanding. This is the path toward peace and confidence and knowing your run.

To know your run, you will need to know your breath. In doing so, you will discover more about who you are. This is simple and basic, just as the teaching promised. You will know what you need to do and how you need to do it. And, in the first few breaths of the journey, you will begin to understand how far it will take you.

What runners have coined "Runner's High" is what science is calling "flow." In both cases, it is portrayed as a fleeting, near impossible task, and you have to be an expert. Then, it may or may not happen…but it does happen.

This teaching, up to this point, has laid out some key reasons why this state is fleeting, why society has trouble achieving this exalted state of being. An overstimulated mind. A mind fed by society to be competitive and fearful, to fight for more—more success, more stuff, more health. A mind hungry for attention and recognition. A mind busy calculating, worrying, thinking, and convincing. An egoistic mind that perpetuates itself. A competitive mind that wants to be better than others. A mind that you "think" is you.

While the mind is magnificent and a part of you, there is more to you and something more magnificent. The mind is at its best when it is at peace.

Peace is not an inactive state. It is a state of the greatest activity, for it engages your life with great purpose and intensity, activating all of your powers and giving them uniform direction. Running is one of your paths to discovering this mystery.

Here is a little secret. Flow can happen and does happen anywhere and at any time. If you are breathing, you can be in a state of flow. You can be sitting, reading a book, and have a taste of the Runner's High. How is this so? The common denominator is having the soul be present. That's it. Allowing your essence to be involved in your action.

Having your soul dance with your mind while tangoing with your body is the secret to obtaining this heightened state of awareness, this state where you feel your best and perform your best, this state where creativity and perception flourish, this state of focus and timeliness and being connected, this state that people have a hard time putting into words…this is your soul speaking, dancing, playing, and being in your life. You will soon know this as Pure Experience.

Pure Experience is being you. Your total Being. You call it flow, being in the zone, "it," "Runner's High," and any number of terms where words fall short of meaning and insight. Pure Experience is a woven connectedness of your body, mind, and soul in union, in harmony, in peace.

It is beautiful. The simplicity of it all. The complexity of our society makes it nearly impossible to find. Where's your soul? It's not part of your impressive technology. It's not in the cars you buy or the food you eat. It is not in the distractions you seek. It is not in a vacation or at the gym. It's not in your goals or your life's successes. It is not waiting for you in some future better self. *It is in you and it is waiting for you to breathe.*

Many people have taken running—one of humanity's greatest gifts—and made it complex. It is not complex. But your deep-down love for running is easy to manipulate, easy to extort for external rewards, easy to make money on selling the complexity of something you already are talented at. Society's gullibility for a quick fix, meaning in a pill, relationship with a thing, and need for connection are so hungry because the world is made out to be complex. The world is not complex. Society has distracted you from your meaning, your purpose, and your true relationships.

Running is simple, but it takes play to do it well. It takes daily play. It takes connections within yourself and with others. The aim of this teaching is the simple joy of running. This is knowing your running. This is knowing your True Self. This is having a Pure Experience.

"The key to growth is the introduction of higher dimensions of consciousness into our awareness."

—Lao Tzu

6b
BREATHING AS A
BRIDGE TO THE BODY

The NightRunner takes opportunities many would use as an excuse not to run and sees them as a beautiful challenge. A prime time to pay attention to the moment and know true compassion. There is only good weather with good gear.

Running at night, regardless of the circumstances, is an opportunity to feel alive and thrive.

SHADOW RISE

Crunch, crunch, breathe. Crunch, crunch, breathe. The rhythmic sounds of your body running through a mountain gulch on snowy trails invigorates the senses. The dusk air stunning in its crisp and lucid panorama has you piercing the universe. Running uphill to the east, the scene bores into the deepest regions of your mind. The pure white silhouette of the mountains contrasting with the shadow rise's purples and blues puts joy in your eyes. And wow, there's even some pink.

Crunch, crunch, breathe. You want more. The timelessness is welcoming and calming. Your eyes scan the cloudless evening sky. Limited in their ability to see everything, your neck cranes back toward the west and again, the joy in your eyes is immediate. The colors are on fire.

Take it all in; soak up the beauty, says your soul. Exhale. Breathe in the world.

The moment-to-moment changes in the brilliant hues of orange and red kindle the heart, while the sun begins warming the other side of the world. Your spirit soars just like your running, and the joy you have been lacking sweeps over you. The stillness—vast and calming— brings nature closer. You merge into the sneaking night.

Running through an orchard, you wonder if the Great Horned Owl is perched somewhere nearby. You wonder if he loves the beauty of this night and murmur this energy his way. Your winged friend recognizes the communication and bellows out hoots in agreement. You smile, mostly on the inside, but the grin is evident on your face as well as in your pace. Crunch, crunch, breathe.

Breathe in the joy.

CONSCIOUS BREATHING

Our first act in this world after leaving the womb of our mother is to fill the lungs up with their first dose of blessed oxygen. You do this with an impressive display of concentration: you cry. Thus, filling your lungs with copious amounts of life-giving air. The rhythmic frequency of life continues to sing with each moment you experience. The first breath you take just might be the "biggest" of your whole life.

Breathing is with You. Where are You?

"Your breathing should flow gracefully, like a river, like a watersnake crossing the water, and not like a chain of rugged mountains or the gallop of a horse. To master our breath is to be in control of our bodies and minds. Each time we find ourselves dispersed and find it difficult to gain control of ourselves by different means, the method of watching the breath should always be used."

—Thích Nhất Hanh,
*The Miracle of Mindfulness: An Introduction
to the Practice of Meditation*

As you dive into the mechanics of breathing and begin the journey of mastering the breath while running, it is important to consider the practice of meditation. Simply put, meditation is an awareness, a path towards achieving Pure Experience. It is the view of this teaching that meditation is as vast and creative as there are humans on the planet. Each one capable of applying meditation in a unique way. Another interpretation of the heart of running can be meditative running. Mindful running. At the essence of meditation is a stillness to the mind, bringing the mind to a state of peace, in a state of focus so the greater presence of the soul can play. If the mind is chattering, or worse, shouting, as is so often the case, the frequency does not allow any reception from above or from within.

So, we begin with the end in mind. To run well you have to develop mindfulness. You have to develop inner calm.

Breathing is really just a cue for this awareness. Being mindful is being present with a beginner's mind. Being present with an open heart. A beginner's mind is a powerful tool, a mind open and ready to receive. A flexible mind that takes in each moment with neutral wonder.

John Wooden, one of the most remarkable coaches of our time, understood teaching the basics. He led the UCLA basketball team to 10 NCAA titles and was named the national coach of the year six times. He was famous for taking his star recruits, kids who could have played basketball anywhere in the country, and in the first practice making sure everyone knew how to tie shoes. He would start with putting on your socks. "Be meticulous, focused, and aware, and do it right so there are no wrinkles." Wooden went on, "Now pull it up in the back, pull it up real good, real strong. Now run your hand around the little toe area...make sure there are no wrinkles and then pull it back up. Check the heel area.

We don't want any sign of a wrinkle about it...the wrinkle will be sure you get blisters, and those blisters are going to make you lose playing time, and if you're good enough, your loss of playing time might get the coach fired." All joking aside, what Wooden was doing was getting his athletes to give themselves fully to the task. When they were tying their shoes, they were TYING their shoes. This primes the person to be ready to give themselves fully to the task, whether that is practice, a game, or life.

Wooden, by going to the basics, was teaching mindfulness, but, while his approach got results, he missed a step: he forgot about *breathing*.

Wooden's already powerful technique could take on a whole new layer with a conscious awareness of the breath while tying your shoes, dribbling, passing, shooting, and rebounding. Here's the thing: Conscious breathing is an automatic upgrade for any activity you are doing. Read that again. If there is one thing you take from this teaching, this is it.

It is a simple concept. You already understand it. You may think you already are an expert—after all, you most likely take over 150,000 breaths per week! You are a master, right? But, in the last week, how many of those breaths did you know? How many of those were optimized breaths, deep breaths, healing breaths, energized breaths, and breaths taken in awareness? "But, wait a second!" you say. "My brain stem and medulla automatically allow me to breathe, so why should I think about it?" First of all, don't think about it, instead be conscious of it. Being conscious of it allows your higher self to optimize your breathing. Second, it's not so much about the breath as it is about having the focus and the concentration to observe the breath. You will find, with practice, that a deeper awareness comes.

Conscious breathing will help you relax while being intent with your action. This is magic. It may seem contradictory, but the best performers know that to do well one has to be relaxed. To run really fast means to be really relaxed. Many will grit their teeth and throw muscle at going fast. While this is part of the evolution, eventually you discover a better way. This is mindfulness. Easy-Fast means breathing well to run well. This is giving yourself fully to the task and allowing your top ability to come forth.

Another understanding of mindfulness is the Chinese symbol that represents the symbol for "presence" over the symbol for "heart." To know and understand your running, you will need to be present with your heart. This simple yet profound act can transform your running and also your life.

Wherever your attention goes, energy flows.

While you are running, and when your awareness is on breathing, there will come a day when one breath—one magical breath—can bring forth the Runner's High.

Have you explored giving attention to your breathing to let the energy flow? Take your next breath with appreciation and feel the energy.

PHYSICAL CHARACTERISTICS OF THE BREATH

With this simple exercise, you can understand quickly how well you are doing understanding the mechanics of your breath:

Stand up and put your right hand on your chest and your left hand on your stomach over your belly button. Take as big a breath as you can and hold it for a few seconds.

❚   Do this with a friend or family member and see what happens.

Which hand moved first? Did your right hand move first and/or at the same time? If so, you are not optimizing your breath and are shallow breathing. The correct mechanics of the breath is to first take an abdominal breath or belly breath. To take your best and biggest breath, the belly should expand fully, then finish the inhale by filling up your chest. In this exercise the left hand should rise and then the right hand. As you inhale, the diaphragm expands, pulling air into the lungs and the left hand rises. When your belly is full, finish the breath by pulling air into your lungs. It is normal for the belly to fall a little at this moment as some air moves into the lungs.

If you are chest breathing, taking only a shallow breath, get excited about the opportunity to improve. If you are already abdominal breathing, you can always obtain deeper levels of awareness, improving your concentration abilities. This belly breathing can be done anytime, anywhere, and will improve everything you do.

Today, take time to enhance your moment and allow yourself

the freedom of three exceptionally aware belly breaths. Do this anytime and as often as you can.

No matter how good you're running and no matter how good you're breathing, you can always improve your knowledge of the breath and, hence, improve your running. You are beginning to understand a deeper awareness with the breath as a catalyst.

Breathing knowledge while running allows for two important doors to be opened and explored in depth. The first door is balance. The second door is timing. Aligning both is your posture. With this as your foundation for exploration, you can build and discover for a lifetime. One of those simple truths: easy to understand and yet so difficult to master.

This connection to breathing, which connects the soul, mind, and body, allows for a deep centeredness. This graceful and relaxed state is an ancient practice in martial arts and the key to strength. Having this balance allows for a higher level of immediate and precise control of the "running body." With practice you will know your running on deeper and deeper levels. This will allow for new abilities to be understood, which only opens more doors for discovery.

Easy-Fast will be one of those "higher" abilities that come with engaged practice.

A paradox for most, going fast means going hard. Not so for the mindful. Going fast means a focused relaxation. Contrasting a supreme effort with absolute calm. There is a Buddhist proverb that says, "It is easy to have calmness in inactivity, it is hard to have calmness in activity, but calmness in activity is true calmness." This is not to say that a maximum effort is not given. But learning to stay calm under maximum stress is an essential skill for any runner. Easy-Fast means a deep and honest relationship with the body, mind, and spirit. Knowing the contrast between times when it can beneficial to go fast versus the times when it might be destructive. The Greek term *kairos* helps to illuminate this aspect of Easy-Fast. It means the right or opportune moment, the supreme moment. Kairos is the moment a door opens and the path is clear, but you must run through the door with force in order to achieve the greatest outcome. It takes wisdom to either "set the stage" for this to happen or to "seize the moment."

Your first task for practice after developing a belly breath is to know your current breathing rhythm. Budd Coates, author of *Running on Air*, has discovered an enlightening pathway to knowing your running and therefore finding more joy in your running. But I contend that *Running on Soul* would be another good title for his book. Not only does this process assist with a physical balance and a stronger, more focused breath, it also helps you practice mindfulness in a fun and engaging way that helps you become vastly more aware. Not just in your running but in your life.

On your next run, pay attention to your current breathing pattern. When are you exhaling? Does it correspond with a foot strike? Which side? Is it always one side? Many are constantly exhaling on the same side. This leads to imbalance. Imbalance can lead to injury and, at the very least, less-than-optimized running.

To be more balanced, practice exhaling on both sides. The pattern for aerobic running is a breathing-five pattern. You inhale for three foot strikes and exhale for two. You simply exhale on the left foot strike and then five strikes later begin the exhale on the right foot strike. With a running cadence of 90 rpm, the breathing will feel fluid and graceful with practice.

At first you will get frustrated after a few seconds of concentration. This is a perfect example of a simple concept that is difficult to master. If you consistently practice, there will come a day when this is effortless. Not only effortless but insightful. You become aware of balance and timing in relation to your posture on intimate levels in the *now*.

It is important to note that your aerobic effort is a wide range from top to bottom. Using a perceived exertion scale from 1 (resting) to 10 (running from a bear), your aerobic effort can be from PE4 (easy) to PE5 (moderate) to PE6 (high-end aerobic).

This empowers you to know everything about your running. Not just your form but also your fitness. You can know the right pace simply from paying attention to your breathing moment to moment with or without technology. If you first breathe well, then you will always run well. Let the breath guide your pace. Most runners keep the breath on automatic and let the mind and other competitors dictate the pace without much concern for the breath—until it's too late.

By allowing the breath to dictate your pace, you can constantly and consistently obtain the balance, power, grace, and relaxation needed to sustain your optimal pace given your situation from instant to instant. This is known at a deep and intuitive level. It does not take an external variable like a watch to look at and analyze. It just takes practice to concentrate on something you do every moment of your life and yet rarely appreciate the depth of its power. This is the ultimate biofeedback tool, and it's built in with a lifetime warranty upon birth.

Many of you do tests to find your fitness zones or levels. This is a worthy and fun practice. However, your fitness at the moment of testing is what is categorically defined. If you are still using those same numbers next week or next month, your fitness may be different from any number of variables. Why let the numbers hold you back or force you to over extend? Again, utilize the numbers, but do not be a slave to the numbers. The numbers are a tool and a method for communication, but by knowing your breath, you have a true foundation for knowing your zone.

The ability to be creative with your running, to be free with your running, to focus precisely on your best form and fitness from moment to moment is empowering you to play. You become mindful in your running. This door is open to you now. Run through it with a beginner's mind and discover your gift.

Picture this. You are a few months into practicing your breathing-five pattern and are just starting to have stretches where it happens effortlessly in awareness. You begin to notice patterns with the arm swings and the hips and the knees and foot strikes. You listen to the movement, you feel the movement and know the instant your timing or balance is off likely due to a breakdown in posture. Today, you are feeling springy and have lots of energy, so you decide to take the breathing-five aerobic pattern to the limit. Thus, knowing your top-end aerobic effort. You pick up your pace and begin breathing deep, holding the five pattern. There can be a subtle urge to breathe more frequently, but you control your effort to coincide with the air you are taking in. You become comfortable with the pattern at the edge of moving to the next pattern, which is a breathing three. You play with your form to eke out more speed while maintaining the same effort. This is magical.

Getting to the "ceiling" of your breathing-five aerobic pattern with effort and then finding efficiency with your form to be more relaxed, more balanced, and precise with your timing will improve your abilities. The insights will be profound.

When learning the five pattern, there are many methods to take. One simple approach is to begin the exhale with a foot strike and know that your next initiation of the exhale will be with the other foot. In this way you are not so much as counting each foot strike but starting to know the timing intuitively. For others it may be easier to start the count with the initiation of the inhale. It is a closed loop. A circle or a clock if you will. The key is that each cycle begins anew with the opposite foot.

You will need and want to spend weeks and probably months with your focus in the breathing-five pattern. Eventually, you will be ready to attempt the breathing-three pattern, which can take you through to your top effort. Budd Coates says there is one more pattern after that, a 1-1-1-2, but that is reserved for a few seconds when you see the finish line or a hungry bear.

With a focused play, the breathing pattern will become your default, and your end goal is to be able to go for a run and know on some level of alertness every breath you take. One breath at a time.

The vast majority of your efforts while running should be in the breathing-five pattern, while recognizing the range of aerobic running from easy to sustainably strong efforts. Doing your speed sessions and races under an hour with the breathing-three pattern will yield powerful results. No matter the pattern you are using while running, being aware of your breathing with an ability to effortlessly optimize not just the breath, but the insight it brings related to balance, timing, and posture is the best card you can play. And guess what—it's a card you are always dealt.

Anytime you start to feel *off*, or the suffering is presenting a problem, it is likely that you have lost touch with your breathing. Simply bring your awareness back to the breath and notice the instant improvement. Part of the magic in an experienced and aware "breather" is allowing for deeper states of relaxation. With a deep awareness of the breath comes a profound level of relaxation, even when running exceptionally fast.

Often, when you start to feel off in your running, it can be traced to a breakdown in your form—an emotional state triggered from an overactive mind or pace. All will be improved and solved with an attentive breath. It is a beautiful thing to thrive by being completely alert in your present moment. The more practiced you become, the more you realize this potential for every breath you take no matter the time, place, and situation. It is an innate ability and gift inside every runner, every person. Yet few give themselves fully to their actions and gain these abilities with mindful practice.

Why is it that such a simple concept is not taught and focused on? A lost art? It is being rediscovered now. Be part of the revolution. Tune in and turn up your concentration abilities. Take it seriously—the same way a child takes her play seriously. This is your life and optimizing it starts with knowing each breath you take. A daunting task for many. That's why an art like running can be a catalyst to self-discovery and becoming a better person. Use an activity you love, like running, and take it to the next level. Start with one simple alert, alive, and attentive breath, then expand.

7
MIND YOUR
POSTURE

Make it a point to run in a storm. Put on some good gear, be wise, and utilize the storm's energy to electrify the air. Embrace the challenge with an inner grin. Some of the most memorable and enjoyable runs you will have will be at a time when most of the world runs for the protection of the indoors.

CONTRASTING

Leaving the confines of a cozy fire, you begin your short run with a lively coolness, with the body urging you to generate some heat. With a cross race the next day, this is a short and sweet primer that gives you confidence heading toward the coast into forceful winds and darkening clouds. If it unleashes all that moisture with the chilly wind, you are only minutes from a warm shower. This assurance lets you enjoy the subtle survival instinct that has flooded your body with hormones. You channel this energy into an alertness.

The wind is working against forward progress, and you find yourself relaxing the muscles of the face that keep wanting to tense up. Scanning the horizon, you brace as the energy from the approaching storm is intensifying. Even though it is a mile away, the rain has sailed on the wind and begins hitting your face with such speed that the drops feel solid. Water acupuncture.

You reach the halfway point and take a moment to soak up the scene and all its splendor with the sea tossing, turning, and churning before you. The vast chaos brings with it an element of order and peace. The dance of movement between earth, sea, and water.

Going first into the wind and then turning around and heading back with the gentle push in your back is like running with a presence. As though you are holding hands with a faster runner assisting you along. It feels like gentle encouragement to relax and run with an ease of effort while still sustaining speed.

As the run progresses, you yearn to feel the heart of the storm's energy, and while the full might did not come, it gives you a taste of the elements. The skies part and the sunlight reveals the deep blues of the universe contrasting the all-reflecting white clouds.

TUNING YOUR INSTRUMENT

As part of tuning the instrument (your body, mind, and spirit) to allow for true harmony while running, posture is key. You will notice as you improve focus in breathing that posture is part of the equation. You will not optimize breathing without posture being enhanced as well. Every time you are fortunate enough to become aware of the breath, the next instant should be moving your body's alignment to be in accordance with the best possible breath.

Picture your muscles like the strings of a guitar, in tune and playing beautiful music. Consider this tuning the proper and neutral alignment. Just like any guitar, you will need to tune the strings often. Once you find the sacred neutral string alignment, the guitar is in harmony and has the potential for wonderful music. If you lengthen or shorten the strings from this centered and neutral position, it doesn't matter how well you play, the sound is compromised from having the best frequency and resonance. It is about using the muscles and connective tissues as lines of pull; this movement should result from knowing the central tuning location. Tune the connective tissue to play beautiful music to perform your action with as much free energy as possible. Breathing is a gateway to knowing these sensations and applying them for sweet music in movement.

By watching the breath, it will be heightened in union with body alignment. For the runner, this allows for balance to be understood and applied at these same heightened levels. Then, and only after attentive focus with a certain level of awareness, can you explore the true depths of your timing in a meaningful way. These are the steps. Each one builds toward developing the next. If you attempt to master balance or timing without an understanding of a mindful breath and posture, then the knowledge base for running is suspect. You are in a position of having to unlearn bad habits. This is often much harder than learning a new skill. If you are an accomplished runner and yet realize your breathing and posture are not ideal, be open to change. Use a beginner's mind to assist in shedding the old programing and unlearning old habits, so that you might learn again the art of running on more "solid footing."

To put this in context: two people (with similar abilities) begin a program with a knowledgeable coach; one is a true beginner and the other an experienced runner with bad habits. The beginner will quickly develop the steps and progress past the experienced runner. Often, the experienced runner is simply applying old habits to new steps. Eventually, he may understand that he must unlearn old programs and belief systems before he can progress with the insight he missed in his first progression.

Another point is that it is never too early to participate with a coach. Often, people feel like they need to get themselves ready before working with a coach, and in this process will often do a couple things that end up working against them. One, they do too much or with too much intensity. Two, they apply the form in a way that will develop bad habits.

It is difficult to run for years and then approach your runs with fresh eyes, especially as you are gaining new insight. Letting go of what you have learned is a process that often takes time, because people put hard work and time into developing the process—only to be asked to try it another way. Many people have a hard time accepting this. Once you can accept the change, there is still the matter of unlearning the physical aspects that are sometimes engrained in a trained and experienced runner.

The progression and the steps are as follows: mindful breathing leads to gracious posture, which brings balance and opens the door to knowing your best timing.

Being in the right space at the right moment in the right mindset. As you progress in your understanding of each step, you will have moments of awe. You will feel it and know it. With more practice, you will be able to take one breath and transition into THE runner. THE runner has merged with the action; there is no person separate from the action; the action and the person have combined into one entity.

Body alignment is defined by Wikipedia as "the optimal placement of the body parts so that the bones are efficiently used, so the muscles have to do less work for the same effect." Here is how the Cleveland Clinic defines posture: "Posture is the position in which you hold your body upright against gravity while standing, sitting, or lying down. Good posture involves training your body to stand, walk, sit, and lie in positions where the least strain is placed on supporting muscles and ligaments during movement or weight-bearing activities." It should also include holding your body upright against gravity while performing an action—like running.

Sound running posture allows you to explore maximizing the characteristics of breathing, balance, and timing. A component that ties all these together is being able to relax. This will allow your efficiency to potentially be realized. Without a centered posture, your running will be exposed as a house of cards being built on shaky foundations. Ouch, this is a double negative.

The runner is utilizing body alignment for stability. With stability the least amount of muscle engagement is required to hold. The more stable you are, the less balance you need. If your posture and stability are a work in progress, certain elements of balance will not be attainable. The progression and the steps are as follows: mindful breathing leads to gracious posture, which brings balance and opens the door to knowing your best timing. To attain it, first your posture and stability will need to be enhanced.

Try a standing assessment to see how your current alignment is. Find your stance that shows dignity while being relaxed. Take off your shoes and stand with your feet shoulder width apart. Every muscle, ligament, and tendon possible should find its neutral position. Play with the pelvic tilt and find the position that allows your gluteus maximus (butt muscles) to be fired easily. In your hips, you will find much of the control center for your posture. Rotate the hips all the way forward and backwards, and then, somewhere in the middle, should be your sweet spot. Your deep-down core muscles surrounding the pelvis will be slightly involved.

Your spine should be relaxed and tall, which shows a prominent chest. The rib cage is held naturally off the normal curves of the

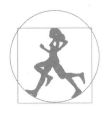

The **progression** and
the steps are as follows:
mindful breathing leads
to **gracious posture**, which
brings balance and opens
the door to knowing your
best timing.

spine. Allow the arms to fall freely from rested shoulders while your neck is beaming toward the sky with a subtle tuck of the chin to lengthen the neck. Tuck the chin to the point where the entire spine feels involved from its base up to your skull. Relax your shoulders and feel like the back of your head is being pulled up to the sky like a puppet on a string. The spine will be true to the sky, not perfectly straight but neutral. Now, turn off all the muscles possible and find a balance that is the most effortless. To hold firm your balance, try to use the abdomen and glutes (butt muscles) to stabilize. Look in a full-length mirror or have someone take a photo of you from the front, back, and side to self-assess your body alignment.

With truly aligned posture, you can remain stable and hold the pose until you need to drink or sleep.

Of major importance with your posture as it concerns running is being able to trigger and fire your gluteus maximus. While standing with your best posture, make sure you can rapidly, easily, and repetitively fire your butt muscles in a squeezing motion. See if you can fire just the right cheek several times, then the left. The gluteus maximus is your best friend when you are running. Unfortunately, many are not even using it for its right purpose. In order to fire the glutes, your posture must be centered; then by applying your balance and timing, you will be able to utilize one of your strongest allies for running power and efficiency.

When posture is balanced and united, you will find that you are also aligned with mindfulness. One of the gifts of being a runner is the intuitive nature of finding a tall and dignified posture with assertiveness. Centering yourself with your individual and dignified posture will allow your mind to be aligned in mindfulness. If you can watch the breath in awareness with a neutral posture, you have laid the foundation for your next steps in your running evolution.

Two aspects of the running code are having the foot strike on your plumb line (dropping a weighted string from the center of gravity to the ground) and allowing the foot to come backwards as it strikes and are directly linked to proper body alignment. Any breakdown in your posture and these elements of sound running are compromised. In one sense, how well you run, measuring stamina and fitness, is directly related to how well and how long you can hold posture. At a certain point gravity wins, but posture allows our batteries to last as long as possible.

To find your true plumb line, you must have your best posture. With this lesson actualized, you can perform striking the ground while your foot is already moving backwards. Being able to strike the ground while your foot is moving backwards is a characteristic of all great runners. Not only is it the most efficient and fastest way to quickly bounce off the surface, it does so with the least amount of impact to the body.

This is the secret to a good foot strike. Many are concerned with a heel strike when they instead should focus on the foot landing on the plumb line while moving backwards. The "bad" heel strike is simply not following the focus stated earlier and landing in front of the plumb line without the foot coming backwards. This is a high-impact strike that is exceptionally inefficient and throws off balance, timing, and posture in one big explosion. Killing six birds with one stone.

If you can find the right posture, allowing for the right balance, you may heel strike on the plumb line with the foot coming backwards and enjoy sound running form with all the speed and health benefits attached. Many elite runners heel strike in this correct manner. (More on the foot strike will be discussed with a deeper awareness of balance and timing in the next chapters.)

Abdominal breathing is one aspect of adapting your best posture. With a chest breath, a runner will stress the shoulders and neck by trying to leverage the spine and lift up the chest for easier expansion of the chest. You will see this with the arms coming up too high when swinging. Not only does this deplete your energy, it also throws off your balance. On top of that, you are not breathing optimally and therefore compromising the oxygen flow to your muscles.

When you belly breathe, you are able to utilize a much stronger muscle, your diaphragm, to breathe. Much of getting a deep breath is the ability to push out the air, thus allowing for new air to reach the farthest areas of your lungs. Beyond just getting a much better breath, you will be more balanced. You will notice an ability to seat your spine in the hips and allow for a relaxed and efficient upper body. Conserving energy and a better flow of oxygen to the muscles means a more joyful running experience—no matter the pace.

These aspects will be discussed further after considering the interdependence of balance and timing.

"A good stance and posture reflect a proper state of mind."

—Morihei Ueshiba

8
THE POWER OF
BALANCE

Discovering the stillness in the night can help you focus on the internal relationships. By aligning the internal relationships, by listening and paying attention to something as simple as your breath, you can drop into a Runner's High.

TRANSFORMING INTO THE NIGHTRUNNER

The night is pitch dark, and as you leave the security of the city lights and enter the void, a rush of the unknown settles into you. At first your eyes have trouble making out anything, but you trust your feet and continue. The emptiness of the space expands your awareness. Suddenly your breathing is amplified and matching a familiar rhythmic pattern with the foot strikes, although new and mysterious in the emptiness of night. Eventually your eyes adapt and the metamorphosis is complete. The NightRunner breathes in the night with heartfelt wonder. Running in the dark, blind to the surface, heightens your balance and you take flight.

The NightRunner is a simple creature who knows there is only great weather with great gear. On this dark and windy night in November, the air is electric with clouds darkening the sky to such a degree as to feel almost completely free. On such a night, the whole world is asleep, but not you—you are awake, as awake as you have been all day.

You reach a spot that you revere and stop. Standing in balanced and relaxed alignment, you observe and listen and smell. High up on a cliff, the crescent moon bay expands before an opening in the trees. The ocean is alive with crashing white water from waves of energy meeting land. The sea breeze brings vast information of its journey and you can taste the salty moisture in the air. You are lost and forgotten; there are only sensory perceptions as time melts away and you are left with an instant of infinity.

You transition from the observer back to The NightRunner.

The light mist turns into a breathtaking storm and the raindrops come down hard on the face. The external energy brings with it an internal energy. You feel it in your pace, you feel it in a deeper connection to life, you feel it in a strong heartbeat, and you feel it in a powerful breath. You express yourself with an instinctual howl. The synchronicity of the instant and its connection is a wonder. You're thriving while contrasting the rest of the world, finding comfort in the coziness of their homes. The wind and rain reach out and touch you in prevailing thrusts of energy. You run as one with the storm and the night. You merge with the emptiness and vastness of the evening, knowing true peace and harmony.

MIDDLE POINT

Imagine a sphere. Put your awareness in the sphere. You can make it as small as you want and as large as a metallic pinball. Now, with awareness in the *orb,* place it in your middle point—your center of gravity—while running with outstanding posture and balance. Make it the control center with all of your energy and momentum in it. Can you feel it, manipulate it, and balance it with awareness? This is one way to use imagination and creativity to expand your understanding of balance while running. For this exercise, consider the orb, sphere, and middle point all as ways of knowing your center of gravity in relation to your action.

Now, imagine your pelvis as a bowl and build a triangle in 2D or pyramid in 3D up to your sphere, which is in your middle point. With sound form, the pyramid is tall and true, while the orb is still, apart from the slightest rotation and rise and fall. The same rise and fall you see with the head of any strong runner. The rise and fall at the base of the pyramid stays perpendicular and level. Center your energy and momentum, while running, in this middle point, and this awareness will gain immediate insight. To add to this, fill up your *bowl* (pelvis) with water. Many people will spill the water in one of two ways. First, by tilting the pelvis forward and *wetting* your shorts or secondly, by dropping one side of the hip (hip dip), usually the hanging hip that is swinging the leg, and spilling out water on the side of your leg. Try to run with a fluidity that does not spill any water.

Depending on your speed, balance, and posture, your sphere will be in the bowl of your hips *floating in the water* if it is low or up in your chest as high as your heart if it is optimized. The top runners will align themselves in a way that raises their balance to its highest potential. This allows for quick and easy navigation of turbulent terrain. With the body aligned in movement, it has many places of reference to act quickly and subtly (grace in the highest order) to correct for changes in terrain.

It is more than a coincidence that your middle point when running well is located right under your heart. Picture this as a stabilizing mechanism to allow the heart to maximize the resonance of its power and magnify your abilities.

How might the orb lie outside of the body? If you fall, the moment of losing your balance, the orb shoots outside of your body. It also will lie outside if, from a standing position, you bend over. Now, your orb will drop and move out of your chest or stomach. Bending over like this with your center of gravity outside of your body will require much more work from your muscles to hold. Often, using muscles that are not meant to support posture for long periods of time.

The goal while running is to keep your sphere high and centered in stillness around your heart. Heart-centered balance. Amplify your power with graceful balance.

Posture has more to do with your bone structure and finding a way to hold a position with the least amount of muscle engagement. Balance, however, is much more nuanced. Balance is the precise firing of a muscle to encourage a masterful manipulation of being centered in movement. This controlled falling, which is known as running, takes incredible balance even if you don't run well. In fact, if you don't run well, the juggling act of balance may even be more impressive, albeit lacking grace. Balance will involve the movement and momentum of running (imagine the sphere) and applying the fulcrum with leverage and torque to maintain the activity with the most efficient firing of the muscles.

Perfect balance while running (controlled falling) is firing a muscle. It is doing little to stabilize you but everything to move you. The best runners skip the "catch" and go straight to thrust. With poor posture or balance, you will require the recruitment of more effort and more muscles to adjust for any imbalances. With supreme balance, the amount of effort you can cut down on is twofold. Not only is every ounce of effort working for you, but none of that effort is wasted on fixing and adjusting improper movement. To amplify your understanding of balance, use simple aspects of your imagination.

The hips will be the focal point. Watch an amazing runner's hips, and you will think they are levitating. Obstruct the view of the legs to make this clear. The hips are solid, hovering in perfect stillness, perpendicular to the ground and yet the running body is putting out great feats of movement and effort. Yes, there is a small bobbing of the hips, the same bobbing you see in the head. Nonetheless, the hips are well balanced and quiet. In this way, they can be leveraged. In the human body, all sound points of leverage come from aligned posture and balance. The final element is timing, which can only happen with a semblance of equilibrium.

Put your awareness back in the sphere, and imagine you are

running with excellent balance with the sphere located in your middle point near your heart. Your x-, y-, and z-axes (depicted below) are all moving in a way to hold the sphere right under your chest in the vicinity of the heart's resonance.

With supreme balance, the sphere is floating in space, inside your body, and hovers in tranquility even while running with great effort. Having this awareness of your middle point will teach you the subtleties of your running balance.

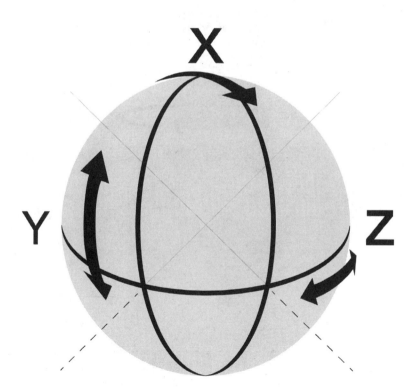

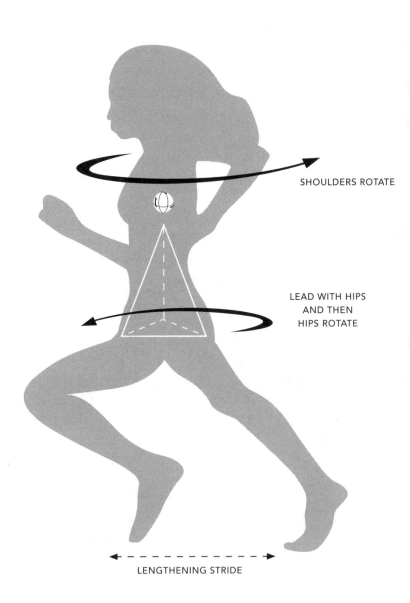

SHOULDERS ROTATE

LEAD WITH HIPS
AND THEN
HIPS ROTATE

LENGTHENING STRIDE

Staying with the pyramid analogy, the base will be rotating. Consider the lead change of the hips as a critical component of torquing and stretching the body with the most efficiency possible. Having the hips rotate lengthens the stride while increasing stability and power by increasing the stretch. High-level running is about stretching not flexing. Tapping into the body's connective tissue and minimizing the metabolically costly effects of flexing muscle (sprinting in events under about a minute require more flex, while endurance events will require more stretch, which uses connective tissue) and having them engaged in just the right way is the key to raising the sphere into the chest while simultaneously shrinking it to the size of a speck. The better your balance, the higher and smaller the middle point. With poor balance, the sphere drops and grows in size.

This enhanced balance of the runner will manifest with a high hip level while running. Measure one's hips when standing. When you run, are your hips lower, the same, or higher? It may be hard to measure hip height while running; a treadmill and slow motion video will help you find the average. Of course, though, this is a trick question, as the answer is all of the above. An advanced runner's lowest hip level is the moment of the foot strike, with a slightly bent knee, and will be a bit lower than when standing. The acceleration and propulsion generated with the foot strike create lift and thrust the hips up. This is subtle, and exaggerating it can be disastrous. However, you will notice a rise and fall of the body with each foot strike. Another way to see this in action is to see the head slightly bobbing up and down.

A runner with marginally off posture and/or balance will

lower his middle point, the result of which is that the pelvis comes down too. With hip height compromised, the runner's optimal foot strike now lies under the surface, literally in the ground. This is only good if you are rototilling the soil to plant seeds. For running it will increase impact and stress on the body as well as require more muscular support to hold the compromised posture. The other end of the scale is manufactured height that creates too much up and down movement and is not showcasing balance.

Stand with dignified posture and feel the middle point somewhere from your belly button to your heart. Now move the sphere around. Note that the slightest change in your posture will move the middle point to a new location.

Many runners keep the sphere inside their body but drop it down into the "bowl" of their hips. The most common is probably the sitting posture while running. Not only does this take the gluteus maximus out of the equation, but the balance is low and the sphere grows in size as it drops to the size of a basketball. You want to raise the sphere, and when it rises, it shrinks down to a point. A well-balanced runner has a speck for a middle point.

To fix the sitting while running, investigate the posture. Go back to the quick exercise of being able to easily and rapidly fire (flex) your gluteus maximus when standing. The slightest pelvic tilt or lean forward from the hips will turn off your ability to easily and readily engage your key running muscles. Not only that, but the breakdown in alignment brings your middle point down and turns the "point" into a volleyball.

Another common mistake among runners is leaning forward from the hips. This can move your middle point outside of your body, which will have devastating effects on your balance, foot strike, speed, efficiency, and stress on the body due to greater impact. The good news is that you will work a lot harder, which is what some people are looking for in running when they are externally motivated.

Envision your running body like a vessel ready for takeoff. Yes, you can fly when you run. A definition of running is simply to only have one foot on the ground at any given moment, and better runners will have no feet on the ground often; flight, lift off, soaring, hovering, gliding, winged, and airborne are all excellent analogies for high-level running. Conversely, the definition of walking is never having both feet off the ground at once, like one does while running. In fact, a great runner is flying.

The better runner you are, the less time the foot is on the ground. You strike the ground in a fraction of a second and then fly through space with supreme balance until the other foot strikes in a fraction of a second, creating perpetual lift.

Your control center for creating balance, leverage, and the power for running lies in and around the hips. A great runner is spontaneously in tune with the hips.

Consider the movement of an airplane and the balance of a runner. On the **y-axis** is the roll rotation or the banking angle. The plane can roll, lifting one wing while dropping the other to assist in changing direction. Unless making a sharp turn, a runner should avoid this movement. However, it can often be seen in runners manifesting with the hips not being squared or level. Your hips are your wings when running, and unless you

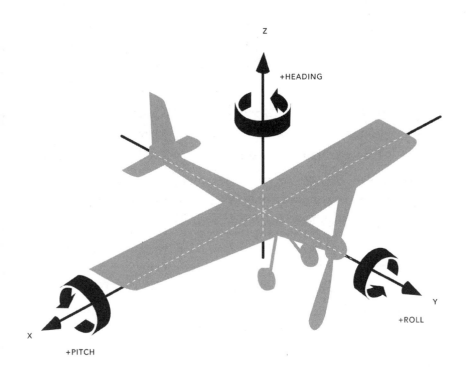

are changing direction, you want to keep them level. It may be helpful to imagine your hips as a flying saucer.

If your hips are level, then everything below and above has a better chance of being in balance. However, if your foot strike is not happening on the plumb line, then this will throw off your neutrality in the hips and hence compromise your power, leverage, and balance. If you are trying to fix the foot strike without first addressing the hip balance, you may never find the sweet spot.

Try this. Stand with your best posture with your feet about the width of your fist apart in alignment with your shoulders.

Notice how easy it is to have level hips. With both feet on the ground, bend the right knee. Notice how the right hip will dip to compensate for this movement. For sound balance, a runner does not want the hip to dip. Conversely, go back to sound posture and keep the left foot entirely on the ground with only the right foot up on the toes. This elevates the right hip, causing the left hip to dip. The only time a runner, like a plane, should use the roll is to navigate turbulence or change direction. Otherwise, the wings/hips are level.

Hip dip is a big problem in the running world. Do not run with a dipped hip. Try this to feel the correct position. Strike your dignified standing pose. Lift up your right leg into your running pose complete with the left arm forward and the right arm back. Have the femur parallel to the ground. The right hip is now your hanging hip. Is it dipping? Imagine and upside-down "L." Your left leg is the long part of the "L" with the short upside-down part being your hips. Keep your hips level. Move the hanging hip up and down, and play with the core muscles that will stabilize a level hip. There is one of critical importance. One that by engaging it is really just serving the purpose of thrusting you forward, but *oh-by-the-way*, it is also stabilizing the entire hip. Do you have the answer? It is where all the magic happens in running…your gluteus maximus, and just your left cheek in this example.

Try it again, strike the pose with your right leg up and flex the left gluteus maximus. Feel the power and the stability. This is how the masters of running levitate their hips; they run with their ass.

Drop a real or imaginary weighted string from your hips to the ground when standing with dignified posture. This is your plumb line. This is the location of the sweet spot for your foot strike. If the foot strike happens behind the plumb line, you fall down. It is hard to go behind the plumb line, and if you manage it, the instant feedback from crashing and burning will make it a quick lesson learned. However, it is common to see a repetitive foot strike that lands in front of the plumb line, outside of it and/ or inside of it. Perhaps the right foot is outside the plumb line, causing the left foot to come inside, for instance.

To fix this imbalance, start with the hip alignment to allow for a better foot strike. Then, you will find more success in altering and improving your foot strike.

On the **x-axis**, the plane will use pitch to change its elevation. For the runner, this is the balance from head to toe. Lean back to put on the breaks and dig into the ground. Lean forward, ever so slightly, and accelerate forward. If done properly, there is a line from the foot up through the head. Many will do the leaning from the hips, putting a bend in the line and hence compromising balance, power, and leverage. This could be viewed by as much a breakdown in posture as it is in balance.

Again, the control center for this balance lies in the hips. But do not bend from the hips when using pitch. Common running lingo is "standing tall," "a puppet on a string," and "straight spine" when speaking about the balance of your pitch angle. While running on a level surface, you should be able to have a straight line from the ground up through your head, and it should be at 90 degrees or just a degree or three forward from the ground. This does not matter if you are running uphill or downhill; you will want to maintain the same angle relative to "flat" ground. If you are running uphill, the angle is sharper relative to the ground, but you should still hold the same 90-degree angle relative to what flat ground would be.

If you lean into a hill climb and make the angle sharper than it already is, you lose balance, placing the imaginary middle point outside of your body and loading up the lower leg, namely the Achilles tendon.

The same applies for running downhill. Find the 90-degree angle relative to what the flat ground would be and hold this angle (unless the angle is so steep that you need to lean back to slow down). Your balance is relative to the pull of gravity, which is straight down to the center of the earth, regardless of going up or down a hill. This is easy to imagine and visualize if you use the puppet on a string analogy and have the puppeteer up in the sky directly above you.

In all cases, up, down, and flat, leaning back will assist in slowing you down, and breaking as your angle relative to the ground will facilitate having the foot strike be in front of the plumb line. Conversely, leaning forward with an almost imperceptible degree changes your alignment (assuming posture holds straight from toe to head) to facilitate landing as far back on the plumb line as possible, creating a situation where you can feel like you are simply falling forward and catching yourself.

The x-axis and the pitch angle are the main balance that creates the bad heel strike that many runners have. If your angle relative to flat ground is greater than 90 degrees, the alignment to the ground is impossible to find the plumb line, and you will foot strike in front of the plumb line. Modern-day shoes assist with padding to enable this technique to continue for some, and with others it will still cause too much stress on the legs, hips, and lower back. Another form of poor heel striking is when a runner, to obtain the forward lean, leans from the hips. This is a breakdown in posture, which moves the middle point sphere of balance outside the body and makes finding the plumb line impossible. In both cases, it is like riding a bike and holding down the brakes. It's great if you want a harder workout, but you will need to replace the brake pads sooner than later.

While it is the foot strike that most see as the problem, they are correct in a sense. The first step in fixing the foot strike is with a combination of posture and balance. Usually, correcting the hips is the first place to look and analyze.

The focus with the pitch and the x-axis is to stand tall with an imaginary line that shoots down to the center of the earth and up through your spine, through the back of your skull and into the heavens. With this posture and balance, you have an opportunity to find the sweet spot for your foot strike. This alignment connects your vessel below and above. Be the bridge that resonates the earth and sky.

On the **z-axis** is the heading and yaw where the airplane will use the rudder to turn left or right. For the runner, this would be a swivel on the spine. In the hips or shoulder, this would be a rotation where one side goes forward, causing the other to go backwards or vice versa. In the foot strike, this is the leverage and power. In order to utilize and/or achieve this balance and the power and leverage that comes with it, you must first have exceptional balance on the x- and y-axis.

This is of high-level importance to conceptualize. Imagine the right foot is at the instant of making contact with the ground. Feel the hanging hip; rotate it as far forward as possible. Now, in an effort to peel off some layers to the onion, imagine the left hip rotated in front of the right hip. Try it if you want from a standing position. Strike the running pose with the left leg up, femur parallel to the ground, and rotate the left hip forward, moving the knee straight ahead. Eventually, you will fall forward. This z-axis rotation of the hips is known as "lead change." It is something all the great runners do whether they are aware of it or not. It can be hard to see, but if you know what to look for, it is clear and easy to incorporate and teach.

Take a deeper look at lead change. On the other side, at the toe off, the hip is rotated backwards. This is actually what you see in a masterful runner. This is how they thrust forward grace and power. This is the leverage to key on. Start here when running, and everything else will have a chance to fall into the right place. The focal point for enhancing this leverage is the gluteus maximus. Your butt supplies the seat, the stability, the balance, the power for true running. Your butt is the workhorse. Your butt is the counterweight. In running, its strength is in acting as a counterbalance to the running load.

The running load the glutes counterbalance has three main points. By tuning into these movements, feeling the interconnectedness, and applying the right balance, a new level of running can be achieved.

This lead change (z-axis rotation) is a key component of what is considered the most gifted and talented runners; it is a magical force for any runner. The key points of the body that leverage this motion are the shoulders, hips, and feet. The hanger shoulder and the hanger hip allow for the arm swing and the leg swing. The hanging hip is involved in the leg swing with the leg off the ground and accelerating forward. While both hips are hanging, consider the opposite shoulder to the hanging hip. Example, the right leg is swinging forward, so the right hanging hip is moving forward with the left arm swing (left shoulder hanger). Note that the upper body arm swing is always opposite the lower body's leg swing. This is a powerful aspect of the z-axis balance that is worth diving into. The hips and shoulders use this leverage to create power, and you want to engage this swivel. The foot strike has the component of striking the ground efficiently and forcefully, but it is also the leverage that goes up the chain through the core of the body.

The contralateral behavior of the runner will use this z-axis balance to achieve efficient and powerful force. Contralateral behavior is how the body is designed to move with the most strength, efficiency, and balance. It can be referred to as the "x," as the focal points through the body end up creating this "x" pattern. Contralateral behavior happens on opposite sides of the spine where leverage, balance, and rotation are used for precise and powerful motion. Consider how the left arm and right leg swing forward together, while at the same moment the right arm and left leg are moving backwards. This contralateral behavior is key for utilizing rotation with the hips and upper body.

This rotation is the power source for running. While the hips are rotating clockwise, the upper body is rotating counterclockwise and vice versa. This torque is powerful.

To understand this in more detail, consider these three key points of focus. When the right foot is on the ground, connect to the left hip, which then connects to the right shoulder. These are points 1, 2, and 3. When the left foot strikes the ground, connect to the right hip, which connects to the left shoulder. These are points 4, 5, and 6. Points 1, 2, and 3 work together in a snap at the instant of the foot strike. They leverage each other in space by resisting the z-axis and holding firm. You can feel this 1, 2, 3, snap, 4, 5, 6, snap for each foot strike, but when you exhale, you will have an elevated sense of the balance. You will notice it happening with each foot strike, but the awareness when you exhale will be a deeper understanding.

Consider points 1, 2, and 3 as yellow and points 4, 5, and 6 as blue. Yellow and blue make green. The yellow points 1, 2, and 3 form one of the "x's" with the blue points 4, 5, and 6 forming the other arm. They intersect to blend hues of green that are your point of balance. The lower "x" balance being at the knees and the upper "x" balance being the middle point or the location of your perfectly balanced sphere.

By tuning in with each breath you take, it will carry over into each foot strike. There is an "x" below the hips from the foot to the opposite iliac crest of the hip. Then there is an "x" that goes from that iliac crest to the opposite shoulder. Only one arm of the "x" is activated and the lower and upper "x's" are always complementing each other.

Feeling this in action will help you love and enjoy running

on a deeper level of understanding with each and every step and breath. Your awareness and focus can constantly grow in this one simple aspect of running. There are many ways to play with this, but the following can provide a path to many others.

Once acquiring a certain ease with your symmetrical breathing pattern, you will notice, on the exhale and foot strike, certain patterns. Patterns that can be leveraged and improved. Start by noticing and connecting the foot strike to the opposite hip. This is one arm of the lower "x" in the contralateral behavior chain. Over time, and with each breath, draw a connection with the foot strike and the opposite hanging hip. The hip that is initiating the leg swing. This grows the myelin sheath, a nerve fiber or axon that facilitates the transmission of nerve impulses. When you learn a new skill, the transmission travels weakly and slowly. With practice you can turn the transmission into a supercharged, lightning fast impulse.

The insight into balance, posture, leverage, power, and timing is impressive. By stabilizing the hanging hip, you provide support and stability for the upper and lower body. This hip serves as a fulcrum for the arm and leg swing. The hanging hip is driving the leg forward, driving the knee forward at the same time the other arm of the "x" on the opposite side of the body is providing the stability from the hanging shoulder for the arm swing.

This is not easy to feel and focus on. At first, it will be a fleeting experience. But you will notice with practice this pattern at the moment of exhale and foot strike. Imagine the knee just like your fist. Now connect the right side with the left, and vice versa. When the left knee is driving forward, the right fist is doing the same thing at the same instant. With the hanging hip and shoulder in a position of balance and stability, you can maximize your efficiency and grace even with high-energy output.

Again, enjoy the process and take it one step at a time...or, better yet, one breath at a time. You will find your focus amplified with each exhale as each exhale will alternate foot strikes and allow for a deeper understanding of the pattern to emerge. At first, simply time your exhale and left foot strike with a connection to your right hanging hip. Then, on your next exhale, feel the connection, balance, leverage, stability, and grace from having the right foot strike and the left hanging hip be in congruence.

While the hanging hip is not rotating, it is still helpful to imagine an arrow shooting forward out of the hanging hip at the moment of the foot strike on the other side. This core engagement is the source of efficient power.

Over time you will notice other aspects of this contralateral behavior that are all working together in crisscross patterns across your body. Eventually, notice that the arrow shooting out of your hanging hip is aided by the opposite side's arm swing, which is supported by the stability and balance of the hanging shoulder at the top of the "x" chain.

In the beginning, it will be best to focus on either the top "x" (the hanging hip to the hanging shoulder) or the bottom "x" (the foot strike to the opposite hanging hip). After a few weeks, your concentration abilities will be at a point where you can feel the upper arm of the "x" contrasting and supporting the lower arm of the "x."

With time you will open up even more doors. Another door

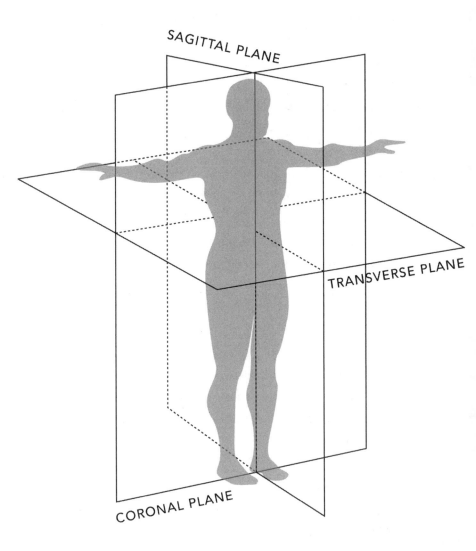

SAGITTAL PLANE- pitch/x 1

CORONAL PLANE- roll/y 1

TRANSVERSE PLAN- heading/yaw/z 1

to explore is the synchronicities of the foot strike. There is the exhale and the relaxing of the diaphragm. The alignment of the top half and lower half aligning at the hips. The legs and the arms are always swinging against each other on the z-axis, and at the moment of the foot strike, the knees and fists meet in alignment. Where both the knees and the hips are crossing each other and lined up on the coronal plane. The power in this moment is using the hips as a fulcrum and feeling the forward thrust from the knee and opposite fist swinging forward.

Now, you can go to higher levels of understanding. To stabilize, leverage, and power this movement at the foot strike, the core muscle to engage is the gluteus maximus—your best friend when running. When the right foot strikes, you engage the right half of the gluteus maximus that is then a tool for torquing and stabilizing from the fulcrum point. Even with just the right glute firing, it will help in stabilizing the left hanging hip. It will provide power working against the z-axis from the foot's placement.

With proper alignment, it utilizes the hamstring without taxing the hamstring. It also allows the quadriceps not to play a role in wasted stabilizing motions. With the upper body, the glutes provide the seat and the support across the body over to the shoulder hang and arm swing.

The glutes are key for balance. They act as a counterweight. That's why they are in your rear. They are large, strong muscles developed for the rigors of impact running. Unfortunately, many do not have the posture and balance required to fire them correctly.

This zigzag pattern of muscle engagement complements muscles from each half of the body. The corresponding of each foot strike is a wonder in balance, efficiency, grace, and concentration. Even when it becomes natural and easy to feel these movements, there is always a smaller middle point. There is no balance, only movement and relationships to achieve with subtle tweaks in recruitment and alignment. There are so many moving parts that you will always find another door to open.

Building on these contralateral movements, the "x" patterns, consider going further and exploring the following scenarios.

Imagine the slingshot runner. See in your mind points 1, 2, and 3. At the moment the right foot impacts the ground, let this be your base leverage for the slingshot. The slingshot is sideways. The leverage of the slingshot is your right shoulder and right foot. The stone that you are going to launch will be shooting out of your left hip. The right shoulder and foot are where you attach the ends of the imaginary band for the slingshot. Then, for the left hip, and at the instant of impact, pull the bands and fire the stone, which will fire out of the left hip. This is essentially a rotation of the hip swiveling against the upper body and creating dynamic movement with powerful and efficient energy. The right shoulder and foot hold their place in space while the left hip is catapulted forward. Picture this as someone holding a slingshot sideways with each point of the Y being the right shoulder and foot. In the middle is where the stone fires. This is the left hip.

A bow and arrow work just as well with the right side shoulder and foot being the tips of the bow and where the strings nock. At the moment the right foot impacts, the bow is loaded and the string is drawn with an arrow ready for flight. Release the arrow by allowing the left hip to fly forward. Imagine an arrow flying out of the left hip. Use the lines of pull to effectively counterweight the body's natural connective tissue.

This *arrow* firing out of the hip is symbolic of the magic in running. The hips being thrust forward with powerful glutes, while simultaneously being torqued from a rotating system. It is a fun exercise to play with to see how many *arrows* you can fire true. Just make sure you are firing them forward and not dropping them from your behind.

These slings are throughout the body often forming these contralateral lines that allow for torque from rotation. Consider the two largest muscles in the body, the gluteus maximus and latissimus dorsi. Now reflect on how the hips rotate opposite the thoracic cage (the rib cage above T12). When the left arm is swinging forward, much of this is created by the rib cage rotating forward on the left. This will stretch the lat. Meanwhile, the right gluteus maximus is being stretched when the right hip rotates forward. Notice the careful choosing of the word "stretch" versus "flex." Here, you have one arm of the "x"- (\) in the contralateral behavior stretched, the left lat to the right glute. In between these two muscles is a lot of fascia, a large amount of connective tissue in the lumbar region. Using this connective tissue for motion is the key. This connective tissue is the rock from the slingshot or the arrow from the bow. Stretch and release the kinetic energy. In this way, you avoid the costly metabolic cost of flexing muscle and utilize the connective tissue.

Your connective tissue is with you while running. Are you using it?

If you can acquire the posture and balance needed to run with your stretch, then you are on a path toward centering your running in alignment with the grand design as read from the User Manual.

Stretch, don't flex, and you will discover running's grace.

Remember the User Manual? The User Manual that came with your body and mind when you incarnated into this world from whatever belief system you have from biology to religion. Oh, you mean, you did not read it? Who can blame you? You open the package in awe, try it on, and start exploring your world, assuming at some point you will come back to the User Manual. But you get distracted. Eventually, you forget that there ever was a User Manual.

So we are left to discover the User Manual through experience. If we work together, we can discover the pages much faster than alone. Alone it would take a thousand lifetimes, maybe more. Together we can read much of the manual in one lifetime. We do this through relationships.

In seeking out relationships, you mold a new key and perhaps decipher a word, sentence, paragraph, or for heaven's sake, a whole page of the User Manual.

We seek experience through relationships to acquire keys to discover aspects of our collective User Manual.

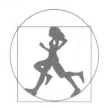

Stretch, don't flex,

and you will **discover**

running's grace.

9
HEALING IS A
CHOICE

Having a Runner's High means listening to the internal guidance system of the heart. The heart does not shout, but its message is loud and clear. From moment to moment, it gives you the best choice. It empowers you to know your truth and to make the decision that sends you on the best possible path. Allow the stillness of the runner—in tune with her breathing and her heartbeat—to know the will of the heart.

AUTHENTIC GUIDANCE

Moon, a waxing crescent, moves on the west horizon toward the other side of the world. With darkness creeping over the land and the running body like a blanket in the silence of night, The NightRunner expands her awareness into the void. Her actions diverge from all those around. Most everyone is inside. Inside small spaces. Few, if any, are outside. Outside in the expanse of night. She is part of the world now, out in nature. Being nurtured by the forces of nature.

While running, the evening feels young, it feels alive, and the darkness contrasts the bursts of starlight finding their way through the clouds. The eyes cannot help but linger on the soft yet energetic light traveling the vastness of space and reaching the eyes mid stride.

the "little me," the will and awareness of the small mind gives way to a deeper presence, a deeper knowing that takes over her Being. The NightRunner takes in the totality of the surrounding environment to an intimate level. The darkness in the wilderness contrasts the moon's soft glow and starlight. The quiet depth of the peace and stillness is contrasting the rhythm of her foot strikes and breathing. The awareness of the "little me" steps aside. The awareness preoccupied with control desires, and improving on the present moment. The little awareness consumed with judging and wanting.

The nature of being outside assists the "little me" with a stillness and a stepping aside for something greater to occur. A higher awareness comes into play, one that empowers. One that can stand the hair up on the back of her neck with an intense love. An awareness with an in-depth connection.

A trained NightRunner enters the will of the heart in the first few breaths of any run. Here lies a deeper awareness. One that accepts the moment, one that is at peace with the moment. A total willingness to surrender to the instant and experience the entirety of one's experience. The NightRunner's trigger is the breath, specifically the runner's breath. But an experienced NightRunner does not stop there. She learns to apply the breath and the will of the heart in many other activities.

The NightRunner first learns to go to a place that is, finally, no longer in an argument with what is. A place within. A place that brings compassion and a stillness that allows you to embrace the ultimate peace. It is the sacred place, and it is inside your heart. ·

A place in ourselves that is no longer controlling and manipulating, a place that lets go, that is not waiting for anything to change or become different or somehow enhance the moment.

The NightRunner enters a dimension of being, a dimension of experience, a dimension of peace, tranquility, and truth, aligned with her true nature: the Heart's Will.

The NightRunner runs with heart and soon discovers a way to live with heart.

SELF-HEALING

In silence you discover this essence deep within you, this most authentic part of you that can taste the air, smell the stars, see the sounds of the owl flying in the stillness of the night, and feel the beating of a heart. Aligned with the breath and the footsteps and the stars above and earth below. Being in this space aligns you with the present moment, and the *Heart's Will* is like your moral compass. This moral compass will guide you towards the best path.

Through the *Heart's Will*, you experience things very deeply and directly. Here, compassion and clarity allow you to make the correct choices, to be aware of what you are supposed to be aware of. You are not running; you are the runner. An empowered soul dancing in the starlight. In touch with such an energy and vitality that the innocence of the universe sweeps over you.

The NightRunner breathes in the awareness, then flexes her awareness muscle out into the stars and beyond.

> *"All healing is first a healing of the heart."*
>
> —Carl Townsend

The heart spark is the most powerful energy in the universe, but you will have to ignite it with your intention. Love is the fuel.

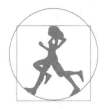

The **heart spark** is the most powerful energy in the universe, but you will have to ignite it with your intention. **Love is the fuel.**

Now that a path has been illuminated for opening the heart and running with centeredness, consider the potential for healing. Healing runs, a run that accelerates and amplifies the healing process. By sensing your body and feeling the rhythm and focusing your awareness, you can open up to higher states of being. With the presence and intelligence of the heart, you can tap into the rhythm, nature, and needs of the body. By understanding and appreciating the body's innate ability to restore and establish balance, going for a healing run/walk can be a most powerful act. The *Heart's Will* may in fact be the most powerful force in the universe.

As you develop meditative attention, the heart will present itself with the natural and innate ability for the body to heal. As you listen, feel, and know the harmony of the heart, you begin to align with its pulse. You are beating to the same drum, dancing to the same music.

The beating of the heart is a vibration that touches every cell in the body. Considering that there are more cells in your body (trillions) than galaxies in the universe (billions), this is a force that will send your body in the direction of your intent. What is your intent and the vibration your cells are aligning to?

Running has many ways to increase the healing potential. One is by simply increasing the energy available to the body. Another is by facilitating the smooth flow of energy, opening up the body to remove blockage and congestion with a general increase in blood flow carrying oxygenated red blood cells. Running can create greater symmetry and balance in the energy field for the body. Running will often get people out into nature, creating one of the marvelous 1 + 1 = 3 scenarios. What!? 1 + 1 does not = 3! Right. But most of the time people think in linear terms or simple arithmetic. When you go for a run to simply increase blood flow + run in nature, it is more of an amplification, like squaring the numbers to have an exponential effect. The combination can be a potent healing potion.

A major force for a healing run is by growing the awareness muscle and applying your intent. This begins a process of aligning an entire universe of cells inside your body. Being able to focus your intent and hone in its abilities will have far-reaching effects on your health.

Science is beginning to understand the nature of consciousness and how it affects our biology. What they are finding is what the ancient teachings have taught for a millennium. That consciousness through pure intent is king. It is, in fact, the environment shaped by your belief system that will dictate much of how your DNA reacts. Your consciousness has much more power to activate your gene expression than anyone has been taught in school. The amazing reality is that your consciousness and its perception send out a signal to every cell in your body. What signal are you sending?

"The moment you change your perception is the moment you rewrite the chemistry of your body."

—Bruce H. Lipton Ph.D., renowned cell biologist and author of *Biology of Belief*

For the heartfelt runner, this is good news. You already know how good running can be for you, even by just mechanically doing it. Imagine the possibilities of empowering your runs to a whole other level.

To this point, the teaching has laid out a foundation for the potential to take full advantage of a conscious running experience. Consider the steps to open up that potential to take full advantage of a healing run/walk. This is at the core of empowered play and gives you the tools for self-healing.

- **Begin** with the self-awareness and intrinsic motivation.
- **Know** the hierarchy and the relationships within (body, mind, heart, and soul), and understand the emotions and the beliefs emanating from these relationships.
- **Love** yourself. You must be kind, accepting, and forgiving of yourself.
- **Find** courage to be able to seek a process of growth and change.
- **Take** responsibility for your actions, decisions, and beliefs, utilizing the support of others but ultimately accepting the role of ownership for your life balance.
- **Take** action by knowing your next best step for self-healing and self-care.

There are many paths that establish a modality of healing. This will be an exploration into running/walking as a self-healing option. Often, people will skip to the last step and take action without laying the internal belief system necessary for profound and lasting change to take shape. While taking action will and does yield benefits, it is weakened significantly if, for instance, you have not come to terms with a deep-rooted love for yourself. To receive the full effect of the healing process, each criterion above must be realized and known. No one but you can accomplish these tasks. While support can certainly help move you in the right direction, it is you who has to take the steps. It is you who will need to open the door and step through.

An important area to consider as part of allowing yourself to honestly love yourself is to forgive yourself and others. Either way, if you are harboring negative thoughts for yourself or someone else, it will be hard for you to progress to the highest states of your ability. Do not carry the sack of potatoes on your back any longer than you need to. To move forward with the grace you are capable of, let go of the added weight. Easy to say, but a whole other action to follow through on. Awareness is the first step in the right direction.

While this is a solo journey, the power of support and love from others is an effect that will move mountains. Giving and receiving love from family, friends, and strangers (and animals) can be the most powerful action in the universe.

INNATE HEALING	TRIGGERING DESTRUCTIVE FORCES
• Growth	• Decay
• Thriving	• Surviving
• Positive challenge	• Negative challenge
• Positive work/exercise	• Negative work/exercise
• Learning	• Overwhelmed/frustrated
• Expanding	• Holding/stagnate
• Healing	• Deterioration
• Love	• Fear
• Recovery	• Loss
• Rest and relaxation response	• Flight or fight
• Absorption	• Breaking down/ overstimulated

Running is a stress, and there are many variables in your control to assure a eustress (positive) response as opposed to a distressed (negative) response.

Looking at the stimulus/response for running can begin with eustress vs. distress runs or positive vs. negative runs. Two people could receive the same stimulus, but one develops eustress while the other develops distress. Even the same person could receive the same stimulus, but on different days it can have two very different responses in the body and mind.

NEGATIVE DISTRESS RUN	POSITIVE EUSTRESS RUN
• Pushing body into prolonged fatigued state	• Absorbed over acceptable time frame
• Too much intensity, overreaching	• Finding right intensity the body can absorb
• Too much duration, going too long	• Finding right duration body will absorb
• Too much frequency, not allowing enough rest between sessions	• Optimizing recovery to grow and absorb between runs
• Poor or incorrect form, being mechanical	• Running balanced and centered, paying attention
• Inadequate sleep	• Resting body and mind
• Inadequate nutrition	• Energizing body and mind with proper nutrients
• Too much life stress	• Balancing life stress

To obtain your desired results with running, you must consider a number of variables. The empowered runner connected to the breath with internal relationships based in trust and transparency will know moment to moment and breath to breath on a deep level what the right pace and intensity should be.

Recognizing the natural ebb and flow of the body and mind is an important internal dialogue to be aware of. The body is constantly sending communication to the mind and vice versa. Many runners will have the mind ruling over the body like a slave. "No pain, no gain" is a common creed for these people. Accepted as normal and even admired in some circles, this sort of training can have a honeymoon phase, where external results and rewards will come. But the honeymoon will end.

This is not to say that you should not challenge yourself, that on some days you will take yourself to new and unexplored realms of pushing the body and mind. But how you view these actions is of critical importance. You may push yourself at efforts that can only be maintained for certain durations, but those explosive bouts of energy can be a thriving display of play at its highest levels.

To thrive at intense efforts and challenges means expanding your abilities to be in touch with the Kairos; the right time. Kairos is the supreme moment or, as the ancient Greeks say, the opportune moment—for things like your timing in running and applying the foot strike, but also for things in life. There will be certain days and times of day when your body is primed for a

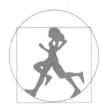

"No pain, no gain" is a common creed for these people. Accepted as normal and even admired in some circles, **this sort of training can have a honeymoon phase**, where external results and rewards will come. **But the honeymoon will end.**

better performance. You cannot simply use will power. You have to recognize the tides. The internal tides of your body and mind. There are micro cycles that are daily and weekly, and macro cycles that are monthly and yearly. Is the tide high or low (equating high tides to big waves and lots of energy vs. low tides with small waves and calmer waters)? Is the tide on the way up or on the way down? There will be days to swim against the tide, but you must recognize the significance of swimming against the current.

When you mirror the challenging efforts with a high tide and are swimming with the current, you will find that your performance is enhanced as well as your ability to absorb and recover from the effort.

When time management is matched up with energy management, then you have Kairos. This is something that thriving elite endurance athletes understand well. You only have so many peak performances. Each one will need to be primed based on a thousand characteristics unique to the individual. It takes some trial and error to discover the limits and know how to prime for your best ability to be showcased. Whether you are peaking for a race or a surgery—or something in between like a business presentation—knowing how best to manage your energy will have far-reaching implications.

Utilizing your energy and maximizing your life force for when it matters most within a day, week, month, and year can be the difference between being effective and being exceptional.

We live in a world that loves to take shortcuts. To be constantly plugged in, turned on, and stimulated to perform whether in business, school, or sport. This creates a high level of burnout. The "I-need-a-vacation" syndrome. This is one area where the best athletes and coaches in the sporting world are light years ahead of the business world or novice athletes and coaches.

The experts of energy management are students of recovery and absorption principles. Stimulus then response then absorb and then repeat. Unfortunately, many are overlooking or skipping the absorption period.

There is a science to recovery, and it is a big deal with a lot of money being thrown at it from many angles. Imagine the advantage a country or federation could have in the Olympics if they discovered an edge for their team's recovery needs.

There is and they did. The British Olympic team had enormously deep pockets for the 2012 London Olympics and the pressure of the entire world's expectations to perform on home soil. "The performance of the athletes has been extraordinary and the collaboration across British sport to make it happen has been nothing like we've ever seen before," said Andy Hunt, Great Britain's chef de mission. Great Britain surpassed expectations by finishing third in the medal count ahead of Russia with 65 medals up from 48 at the 2008 Beijing Games.

Their secret? Recovery. Doing the small things correctly can be the difference when microseconds matter. Incremental gains lead to profound performances. In other words, doing the simple things within our control really well (not to say that is easy—

simple things take a lifetime to master) can lead to the thriving we all seek in our lives.

The British performed many tests to figure out how hard they could work their athletes and yield results. One system stood out above the rest. RestWise. A simple online algorithm that takes just seconds to implement and has better results than invasive lab tests to determine an athlete's energy levels. You simply track some weighted variables, and the algorithm learns your traits and gives you a score from 0 to 100. It then empowers you to adjust the day's training based on the score.

Quantifiable: resting heart rate, hours slept, weight.

Subjective (on a three-part scale of worse than normal, normal, better than normal): How well did you sleep? Describe your energy level? Describe your mood state today?

These are variables well within your control. With awareness of these aspects, you can begin to optimize your day-to-day energy needs. But also you will recognize that even with optimizing these variables, there are still subtle fluctuations seemingly out of your control. Recognizing where on the sliding scale of energy you are minute to minute, day to day, week to week, and month to month is a huge part of the understanding.

Recognizing these variables empowers you toward optimizing your energy. On a larger scale, energy management is about setting the stage for a peak performance when it matters most and allows for periods of absorption and recovery going in and coming out of a peak performance. No one—not even the most talented among us—can maintain the top level all the time. While it might appear that way, to those most aware, they are simply flawlessly priming the body and mind for the peaks and valleys and choosing when they are doing it.

While initially this tool was created for the elite endurance athlete, the implications are far reaching. At the other end of the spectrum, you have people coming out of surgeries and cancer treatments and looking to understand their new levels of energy. The variables have all shifted after and during a stressful life event. When dealing with a serious injury or illness, understanding what is under your control for recovery and absorption is key to getting back the thriving energy levels you once enjoyed and can again.

If you want to set the stage for optimizing your energy levels (which ties into time management too), paying attention to the variables you can regulate will contribute to being your best self. If you are regularly compromising your sleep, then you will not, no matter what you do, be able to find your best performance in anything you do.

At the basis of this RestWise tool is listening to your body. Knowing the internal dialogue between the body and the mind. Having an honest assessment is critical. While the body serves the mind, the mind's command of the body should be one with the utmost respect and love and treatment for a body that is thriving. Unfortunately, many in the fitness world do not appreciate this, and the mind is dictating to the body without much feedback from the body. In other words, the communication is one sided.

This is an empty relationship void of purpose and will have consequences for both the body and mind.

In a truthful and thriving body/mind relationship, the mind is making choices that allow the body to get the sleep, nourishment, and peacefulness in between cycles of movement that can be challenging. In this way, you can improve and learn and grow.

By optimizing your energy management, you can fulfill your time management. By integrating these, you can allow the body and mind to thrive. This is healing at its finest. It is a choice. A choice born from being aware.

10
THE BEAUTY
OF TIMING

Know your purpose when you are running. Simply be the runner. The breath, the blood flow, the movement aligned with one purpose: to run. This is simple; it is not easy. Run with purpose and you will know your truth.

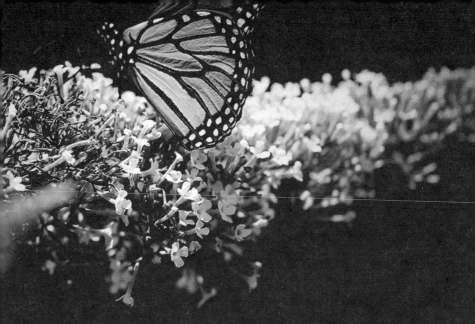

KAIROS AND TRUTH
IN MOVEMENT

Your eyes are open to the low vibrations of a soft dawn. In this moment, you take control of the reins. With appreciation and focus, you inhale the world around you and exhale yourself back into it. You resonate with the space and feel, look, smell, taste, and hear the force merging with each breath. As you make your bed, you let a glimpse of the day enter into your mind. You run almost daily but often do not plan ahead the specific time. Rather, you wait for the Kairos to tell you when to go. By tuning into each moment and listening to not just your body, mind, and soul, but the souls of all those around you. In stillness you can receive the Kairos, the supreme moment, the time to act. In this moment, the soft hues of pink, purple, and a touch of orange are asking you to come. Come out and play. Come now.

You begin with that first footfall and exhale. The transformation is complete. You are the runner. A completion of form with every cell in your body on the same frequency. A vibration known as running. The heart dictates the frequency. You allow the body and mind to follow its lead. It goes much deeper than the heart beats. While the beats are the music for the dance, the heart is also resonating a far greater energy. An energy that aligns your whole Being. It is an electromagnetic pulse. An EMP. An energy that resonates not just inside but outside your body. It attracts what it reflects. It aligns you with purpose when it is amplified. In this instant, you feel a connection with the earth below and the sky above. Your running body a bridge into the unknown. Each moment a new and exciting experience. Inhale the world, exhale yourself back into it.

*You run with passion. You run with the force of your entire Being. You align the universe within to one common purpose. Aligning the trillions of cells inside you with one single focus. In this moment you run, let your whole Being be the action. **Let the whole Being (body, mind, spirit) be in unison and act/ focus on one motion.***

SOUL OVER MIND

If you have followed and used your imagination and practiced and understood the steps to this point, then you have felt, or perhaps witnessed is a better expression, the power of Being the runner. If you can "set the stage," then to Be the action is to be love. It is simple. If you love your action like you can love running, and can be the action, then what are you? Are you the running lover, the loving runner, or merging into the RunLove/LoveRun Being? This is the heart of running.

Science is only now beginning to understand the genius of the human heart. A pump? This is only a mechanical view of something so much more awe inspiring than a mere pump. This only scratches the surface. This organ, at the middle point of the human being, is the marvel of the world. You know what the energy of the heart is; you already know it deep down. You have felt it and it is your strongest force.

The heart has an electromagnetic field that is many times stronger than the brain. The heart has an intelligence beyond what you have been taught in school. If you can create a coherence with the brain (stillness) and receive the intelligence that resonates from the heart, then you can align your form with the moment.

By aligning in the moment, you may experience flow, the Runner's High, being in the zone, and the Pure Experience. In this state of awareness, you can, in essence, slow down time. Your awareness of the moment, a deep understanding and concentration on the present moment, allows you to download more information.

Being aware, being present, being in the zone, all internal organs relax and open up; our focus moves to a broadband state where we can experience much more information. Time slows down. Time slows down because more information is being processed in the moment. In a flow-like way, this is being in a state of flow. A magical time where everything comes up roses. The right information comes to you. You are more quantum-level attuned to a universe of energy. This is where the practice of mindfulness can lead you. The gateway to this realm is a calm mind in tune with the vibrations of the heart.

This is the beauty of timing.

The right timing cannot be achieved until the previous steps have been taken. It takes experience and years of practice to be ready to know the timing. There are many paths to get to this point. This book started with the breath and moved along to posture and then balance before arriving at the holy grail of running: timing.

Timing is more than firing the muscles at the exact instant to propel the body. This is the timing involved with the mind and body. This is mind over matter. Consider the soul over mind for the deeper and higher level of timing. There are clues throughout this book in ways to attain and open this gateway, which lies in the heart. Running is a potential beautiful path to take for this exploration.

In your training, in your learning to learn, notice both aspects with each step. One aspect is the mind over matter, and another is the soul over the mind. You can become physically accomplished as a runner, but this will be a hollow accomplishment if you are just a fit runner and don't have a dialogue with your higher self. True meaning and purpose are accomplished with soul over mind understanding.

With practice you go beyond thinking about your running, beyond feeling your running, into the realm of knowing your running. This is running with heart and soul. It is not limited to running. It can be done with any action. If you are breathing, you can know your action.

In this way, in every action you take, in every action you practice, you can know a deeper understanding.

True understanding is just an awareness, the simplest and yet most profound awareness you can have.

An entire book can be written on the timing aspects of running. Here is a path to know and discover through experience:

Imagine the six key points for running balance. Points 1, 2, and 3 (right foot, left hip, right shoulder) and points 4, 5, and 6 (left foot, right hip, left shoulder). With each foot strike feel the yellow points activate, then the blue points activate. Then feel the lines where they cross and intersect. Yellow and blue mix to make green. Feel these green points; amplify them with each foot strike. One is centered between the knees, and the other is centered in your chest. Let these green points drive your balance and your timing, counterbalancing each side of the body.

You can connect the green middle points to create a third alignment that will be the center of your pelvis.

Now, slow down time by knowing the connection with only

the foot strikes that coincide with the breath. Activate your yellow lines and your blue lines only on the exhale to create the green middle points. This keeps your body aligned and tight in a relaxed way. If one point goes too far or does not engage, the whole chain is thrown off, and you can feel it immediately.

Feel the slingshot with the yellow breath. Launch the imaginary stone from the left hip using the right foot and shoulder as the leverage. This arrow represents the forward momentum of the hanging hip. The hanging hip is parallel to the engaged right glutes that are cracking the whip with the right foot.

Picture the engaging of the right cheek glutes and the cracking of the whip with the right foot as a means to sling the guide wires and encourage the forward thrust for the opposite side of the hips.

Now, move your awareness to the next cracking of the whip, which will initiate from the hanging hip, currently, your left side. This hanging hip acts as a swing for the lower leg. The left knee reaches its climax in alliance with the right fist pump. With the knee at its climax, the lower leg finishes the momentum and extends the leg a few degrees short of being straight. The same sort of action you see with leg pumping that kids and adults do when they are swinging at a playground.

The hanging hip that is swinging the leg forward is also the lead change and rotation (yaw) of the hips. When the knee is at its climax with forward motion, the same side hip is rotated forward. Poised to begin rotating backwards, assisting the foot strike with a graceful backwards thrust. This is part of you activating your spinal engine.

With a good pace, at this point, you are a flying saucer. Airborne, with both feet off the ground. This is when you initiate the cracking of the whip.

When cracking a whip with your hand, it is a flick of the wrist that finishes the acceleration. In this case, the movement that accelerates the whip to crack (your leg) is your glute. The instant your leg finishes its forward swing is the time to engage the left glute. This accelerates your leg to the ground and recruits the firing of the muscles down the chain of the left leg. Starting with the hamstring and moving to the ankle and finally the left foot.

With impeccable timing and balance, your leg accelerates backwards against the momentum of the hips and the body moving forward. The leg whips with the impact to the surface. This engagement is the precise timing to create the most force off the ground. A force that is gentle on the body when the timing and balance are true. A force the human body is designed to thrive with. A force that with practice saves energy by turning the muscles on for an electric instant and then allowing them to relax.

Just like the crack of a whip, the force is quick and powerful. C-r-a-c-k! The thrust boosts the momentum already in progress, and the flying saucer continues its antigravity movement.

In this way, you might feel the lead change of the hips as a passing of the baton from the yellow to the blue side. The height, the stability, and the momentum are sustainable depending on your pace, fitness, and awareness. Often, the first thing to go is the height. You will feel the passing of the baton come down, almost imperceptibly, but it throws off your balance and timing in such a way that the crack of your whip is more of a dull thud against the ground.

Another path to explore was mentioned briefly in the previous sequence. The beauty of a runner in motion and the counterbalance being played out with contralateral behavior is fun to discover and amplify.

Consider the significance of the hanging hip and shoulder. They work together on opposite sides of the body to create wonderful timing and balance. At the moment of the foot strike, the knees and the fists come to their closest proximity as they both cross paths, going in different directions at the apex of their pendulum swing. This is a great place to start each cycle fresh with a new awareness. High noon on the closed loop of the running body cycle starts at this moment when you strike the ground and exhale.

On the yellow exhale, notice the left knee and the right fist (both swinging from the hanging position of points 2 and 3) swinging in tandem in the same forward direction. Play with this action only on the yellow and blue exhales. Feel it working for you with efficiency. Also notice how the timing and balance of one affects the other. The running body is a closed system, and by tuning into each aspect of the yellow chain of movement in contrast to the blue chain of movement and mixing the green points of balance, you can know your run timing on intimate levels. And you know them as they happen—instant feedback.

One other aspect to explore is the cadence and the power of 3, 6, and 9s in running. It is well known that an ideal cadence is 90 reps per minute (one foot strike or 180 if you count each foot), the same for biking and walking. There are exceptions for going faster and sprinting as well as going up or down hills, but generally, whether you are going easy or fast, you want to be at this 90 rpm. Count one foot for a minute to find out your cadence. As you get better and more familiar a short cut is counting one foot strike for 10 seconds, if you get to 15, you are in harmony with the correct frequency. This creates a rhythm you should know by heart. If you are running in the aerobic zone and breathing the five pattern, this is 36 breaths a minute. You will be taking a breath every 1.6666666 seconds. Another way to look at it is that your right foot exhale will be every 3.33333333 seconds just like your left foot exhale. It is a pleasant frequency that allows for a deep and fluid breath.

If you are running at a tempo or higher pace and utilizing the breathing-three pattern, then you are taking a breath every second. Sixty breaths a minute or 30 with each foot. Maybe running has more to it than meets the eye. Perhaps your running body is truly a frequency of divine proportions when amplified correctly.

Nikola Tesla said quite inexplicably, "If you only knew the magnificence of the 3, 6, and 9, then you would have a key to the universe." Ha, well, yes, he was talking about running.

The goal for your running form is to tune into each exhale. By tuning into this vibration, with practice and awareness, your focus will reveal the mysteries of running. You might even reveal the deeper mysteries lying within you. How many breaths can you tune into when you run? How long can you sustain your focus? Challenge yourself and the potential for growth will be endless.

It is exceptionally difficult to pay attention to all the rhythms and motions while running. You may focus directly on one or two aspects of the whole body's movement. Amplify this concentration and know the feeling intimately by knowing the breath. Here, one or two motions that have thousands of angles to discover can be fresh and new even though you have done it 10,000 times. By tuning into the breathing pattern and particularly the exhale, you can expand your awareness. At the exhale, the ground force reaction is being played with rotations within rotations, and for a brief instant, you can know the right foot strike and exhale and then the left, and so on, and so on.

Take a beginner's mind approach to each breath, and your running will forever be one of the most exciting actions you can do. You will continue to work and grow in some aspect of your form, which at its highest levels always comes back to the heart.

EXPLORING THE MYSTERY AND WEIGHING THE PATH'S HEART

A secret link. Flow, play, and mindfulness. At the essence of each is Pure Experience. An experience felt from the heart. At the core of being YOUrself. "Knowing thyself" and discovering your true abilities and your true gifts happens by bringing these states, flow, play, and *heartfulness,* into synthesis with any relationship. When the body, mind, *heart*, and soul are aligned and in harmony, we use terms like play, flow, and mindfulness to communicate the experience. The secret is that these states are really the same thing and all are well within your abilities to attain with this breath. Exhale, breathe in the world of wonder that exists in you now. Do it while running and feel the exhilaration of being alive with your full capacity. Then realize that this exalted state is not limited only to running. You have simply peered through the window of possibilities. Your true potential is in every breath you take.

UNVEILING THE GREAT MYSTERY

At this point, with attention and practice, you are in a position to have a deeper understanding of the mystery. The deeper mystery of this teaching. Running is simply one tool of any action to get at the heart of the matter. Your existence and the greatest question you can ask yourself is, "Who am I?" The hierarchy: the body is action and serves the mind, the mind is thoughts and serves the heart, the heart is emotions, and its most powerful resonance is love. In this way, the heart serves the soul.

You will notice a new revealing in the hierarchy. A critical component overlooked and underestimated in society at large. The heart is the true master, the heart and its ability to amplify the most powerful frequency in the universe: love. It is not so much mindfulness as it is heartfulness. But it takes a certain level of understanding to be able to accept and know this as truth. Certain steps in your evolution will have to be reached before this awareness can be amplified and known.

If you just had an "aha moment," you realize that the right place to start is from the heart. Initiation begins here. Do not "think" that you should initiate from the mind. This is analogous to trying to obtain solid balance while running but having poor posture. Your true balance will never be realized. Not until you improve your posture. Then you may begin with the nuances of throwing your balance; there is no position, only movement when running. If you don't align the body and mind, you won't be able to realize the deeper components of your balance. You have missed a step and therefore may never realize the lesson. To know who you are, to reach your potential, to find fulfillment, to build meaningful relationships, to serve your purpose and quench a deep-down yearning in everyone...you must initiate from the HEART.

Review what you have learned in your "mind's eye" (with a deeper understanding of what was just revealed, you can see how the language that you speak can blur the true meaning), which if you have taken the steps, acquired the keys, and opened the doors through diligent practice and focus, you will actually know this as your "heart's eye." If you read this book with the understanding like most that the mind is the "top of the pyramid," consider reading it again and substitute mind for heart in those circumstances.

The gateway and the portal to the soul are through the heart.

Your true power lies in the ability to first amplify the emotion of love. Any emotion comes before thought. Thought is just a rippling across the mind of certain emotions. This is the lesson from acquiring a still, peaceful, and calm mind. To simply be aware of this aspect of who you are. Run in ~~mindfulness~~ heartfulness. If you run because you love it, if you run to play, if you run to build relationships, then you can practice your gift. Your gift is heartfulness in each breath.

The progression: mindfulness leads to heartfulness to know

yourself and build relationships internally and externally. This will help you discover meaning and purpose. Serving others in teaching/learning and learning/teaching relationships will give insight to further evolve not just in running but in being a better human. Breathing will be the bridge between the metaphysical and the physical realms. This link, this interconnectedness of your Being through breathing, is your cue to complete awareness in this moment. Sound breathing leads to a harmonized posture. With your body aligned and in tune, the middle point can be known and felt for supreme balance. Now, with the previous steps learned, timing can be displayed and expressed with all its grace.

With total awareness of your action, a most pleasant, wonderful, and surprising door is opened. A resonance from the heart. And therein lies the deep mystery and the heart and soul of running or any action. The power of emotion. Realize that emotion comes before thought. To express yourself, run with heart. Center your attention on the resonate qualities of the heart and amplify the love, then express yourself in the action of the moment. You see, your bigger mind is the heart. When you still the mind to receive a greater presence and a greater knowing, this portal is opened through the heart. This is the gift; this is the birthright of every human. To know and express the resonate qualities of the heart.

Love is with You. Where are You?

To run with mystical awareness and feel this joy work its magic on your soul is the gift. This is the essence of running. This is the essence of you. To get to the heart of the matter, start with the body and find alignment. Then go to the reflective pools of the mind that mirror the world for the heart to act. This interconnected synchronicity of your whole Being (the body, mind, heart, and soul complex that is you) finds a balance and a centered awareness that amplifies YOU. This power of the heart, echoing its strongest emotion, is clarity, harmony, and knowledge expressing the soul. This is the power of love. Love your running; love yourself. It is not a very big leap to then find ways to love the world.

When you love yourself and your actions, you open up a world of understanding and empathy for the whole planet. This is the heart of running. Run with truth. Run with heart. Run with awareness.

COMPLETING THE TRANSFORMATION

Wherever attention goes, energy flows. Grow your attention and grow your energy. Use your internal guidance system to be in the moment. Appreciate the sounds of your running, your breath, your foot strikes, and heartbeat mirroring the external world and the stimulus it brings. You can know every breath you take. You can love every breath you take. Each breath can have a knowing to it that has you feeling connected. An expansive connectedness that starts inside and envelopes the whole world. If you can have compassion for your running, you can have compassion for yourself. With this as your foundation, with compassion guiding you, you are aligned with your purpose. You are running with heart. Now live with heart. You have the key.

NIGHTRUNNER'S CODE

*The breaths click off in
the familiar pattern of
1.6666666 seconds as
the count reaches 720.
The NightRunner is on
a 1,440-breath run. Seven
hundred twenty breaths out and then
720 breathes back in a comfortable breathing-
five pattern. This works out to be a 40-minute run.
The bread and butter for The NightRunner's
prowess. With the sunset's low glow
illuminating the hills and flickering
the aspen leaves, a pause feels
like the right action for the
moment.*

*Standing in stillness, the
scene encompasses a new
awareness. The Heart's Will, the
compass that guides the best choices, is
loud and clear when the runner pays attention. When the
runner becomes aware of being aware. The expression
that can be felt and known expands into a new dimension.
When the runner runs, all those problems and worries
melt away if only for a moment. Herein lies the beauty.*

The first stars appear in the sky and The NightRunner casts a glance towards Jupiter. The Heart's Will says it's time to run again, and the first strike to the ground is met with the awareness of 721. Five steps later is breath 722. Each breath has a depth to it. Not just an awareness within but an awareness surrounding her Being.

The NightRunner knows life is all about relationships. The relationships within, the relationships with her external world, the relationships with people. These are the experiences that allow her to evolve and grow. These relationships are the only thing she holds forever.

The NightRunner's heart is beating to a singular pulse resonating throughout the whole body. Truth is known. Alignment is met. The internal guidance of the heart is felt and listened to. The true runner is a whole-body heart running. Each cell in the body pulsing to the same beat, all with a singular purpose.

A certain frequency is met. An electrical spark of thought mirrors a magnetic emotion. It is the most powerful electromagnetic pulse in the universe. It is simple. Yet profound. The thought? Love. The emotion? Love. It is a choice. A choice The NightRunner amplifies with precision.

The NightRunner learns to be grounded and centered while running, and then the master learns to apply this amplified thought and emotional relationship to any activity that requires a breath. Here, compassion is known.

This is the heart of running. Making the choice.
Being aware. Aligning your thoughts with your emotions
and breathing deep. Holding this space of the heart.
Expressing, giving, and releasing your love into the
world. It can be as simple as loving your running.
Taking a breath, taking a step in awareness.
Paying attention to the internal guidance
system of the heart. The heart knows your
best choice from moment to moment; it
allows you to be in the moment with a
depth of joy.

The night is alive with stars as breath 1440
is taken, and The NightRunner transforms from the
runner to the walker and yet continues to enjoy full
consciousness, a fully aware state that is familiar and has
a sense of ease.

ABOUT THE **AUTHOR**

The Heart of Running is a love story born from a relationship with the self, family, and friends. Kevin enhanced this journey of exploring these potentials when he married his wife in the Sawtooth Mountains of Idaho. Sharing the adventure and having an equal to learn/teach from and with has accelerated the evolution of life. The rich experiences from this harmonic convergence allowed for a greater awareness to take shape. Shortly after marrying Hortense, Kevin embarked on a decade-long journey of discovering flow states as a professional triathlete. During this time he also worked for the community through the YMCA coaching all ages and abilities to appreciate the joys of movement. These relationships (relationships are the key) opened up the doors toward understanding deeper levels of awareness not just in athletic performances but in achieving life happiness.

Running with heart evolved into living with heart.

THE HEART OF RUNNING

Kevin Everett is an empowered play expert. He is a coach, mentor, and writer for thriving, wellness, and performance. He is the son of a coach, and so began a lifelong application of being a student. Always curious and grateful to learn from a string of mentors over the years, this curiosity revealed deeper understanding.

Kevin participated as a professional triathlete racing internationally for over a decade while also coaching the joys of this type of empowered play. As much as he tried to teach, he learned just as much. Coaching at the YMCA provided a rich experience and a perfect community center for engaging in best practices.

He loves to explore human potentials by engaging relationships in learning/teaching experiences. He is in his third decade coaching every age and every ability level and enjoys the unique puzzle of each individual's best next step. Kevin has been blessed with great mentors throughout his over three decades of competing at the highest levels in endurance themed events. The feedback loop of being both a coach and an athlete proves to be insightful.

A successful collegiate swimming career earned four NCAA II National Swimming Championships.

After a seven-year hiatus from focused competition (gaining 50 pounds), at 28 he jumped into his first triathlon. He became a professional triathlete shortly after and learned to juggle the love affair already established with swimming, with biking and running too. Running did not come easy at first. But in this struggle was a mighty lesson. It took expert coaches and lots of trial and error practicing to find the joy in running. This struggle helped to instill a deeper appreciation and understanding for running. A little over 10 years into the sport, a culminating moment was achieved when Kevin ran a 32 minute 10k to cap off an LA Triathlon victory celebration at L.A. Live.

With his best years and races still in front of him at a youthful

40 years of age, life balance and the next best chapter in life reflected taking a step back from the demands of competing professionally. The joys of being a father of two young children are pulling him toward new and exciting paths. Learning daily from his kids, the true experts of play, is touching the heart of life. Being in tune with this pulse is the key.

The lessons from competing with the world's best triathletes while simultaneously coaching with the community through the YMCA taught him valuable lessons on a daily basis. It proved to be a rich environment for gaining experience. The gift of working with so many and learning from each person is a gift he wants to share.

"C'est en donnant que l'on reçoit."

For it is in giving that we receive.

—Francis of Assisi

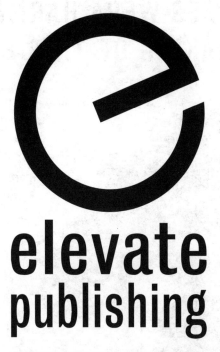

elevate
publishing

DELIVERING TRANSFORMATIVE MESSAGES
TO THE WORLD

Visit www.elevatepub.com for our latest offerings.

NO TREES WERE HARMED IN THE MAKING OF THIS BOOK.

OK, so a few did make the ultimate sacrifice.

In order to steward our environment, we are partnered with *Plant With Purpose,* to plant a tree for every tree that paid the price for the printing of this book.

To learn more, visit www.elevatepub.com/about

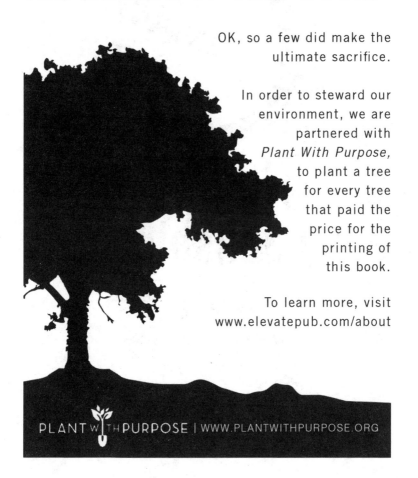